Integrating Federal Statistics on Children

Report of a Workshop

Board on Children and Families • Committee on National Statistics

Commission on Behavioral and Social Sciences and Education

National Research Council • Institute of Medicine

NATIONAL ACADEMY PRESS
Washington, D.C. 1995

NOTICE: The project that is the subject of this report was approved by the Governing Board of the National Research Council, whose members are drawn from the councils of the National Academy of Sciences, the National Academy of Engineering, and the Institute of Medicine. The members of the committee responsible for the report were chosen for their special competences and with regard for appropriate balance.

This report has been reviewed by a group other than the authors according to procedures approved by a Report Review Committee consisting of members of the National Academy of Sciences, the National Academy of Engineering, and the Institute of Medicine.

The National Academy of Sciences is a private, nonprofit, self-perpetuating society of distinguished scholars engaged in scientific and engineering research, dedicated to the furtherance of science and technology and to their use for the general welfare. Upon the authority of the charter granted to it by the Congress in 1863, the Academy has a mandate that requires it to advise the federal government on scientific and technical matters. Dr. Bruce M. Alberts is president of the National Academy of Sciences.

The National Academy of Engineering was established in 1964, under the charter of the National Academy of Sciences, as a parallel organization of outstanding engineers. It is autonomous in its administration and in the selection of its members, sharing with the National Academy of Sciences the responsibility for advising the federal government. The National Academy of Engineering also sponsors engineering programs aimed at meeting national needs, encourages education and research, and recognizes the superior achievements of engineers. Dr. Harold Liebowitz is president of the National Academy of Engineering.

The Institute of Medicine was established in 1970 by the National Academy of Sciences to secure the services of eminent members of appropriate professions in the examination of policy matters pertaining to the health of the public. The Institute acts under the responsibility given to the National Academy of Sciences by its congressional charter to be an adviser to the federal government and, upon its own initiative, to identify issues of medical care, research, and education. Dr. Kenneth I. Shine is president of the Institute of Medicine.

The National Research Council was organized by the National Academy of Sciences in 1916 to associate the broad community of science and technology with the Academy's purposes of furthering knowledge and advising the federal government. Functioning in accordance with general policies determined by the Academy, the Council has become the principal operating agency of both the National Academy of Sciences and the National Academy of Engineering in providing services to the government, the public, and the scientific and engineering communities. The Council is administered jointly by both Academies and the Institute of Medicine. Dr. Bruce M. Alberts and Dr. Harold Liebowitz are chairman and vice chairman, respectively, of the National Research Council.

This project is supported by funds provided by the National Research Council and the Annie E. Casey Foundation.

Library of Congress Catalog Card Number 95-78856

International Standard Book Number 0-309-05249-1

Additional copies of this report are available from:

National Academy Press, 2101 Constitution Avenue, N.W., Box 285, Washington, D.C. 20055. Call 800-624-6242 or 202-334-3313 (in the Washington Metropolitan Area).

Printed in the United States of America

BOARD ON CHILDREN AND FAMILIES

COMMITTEE ON NATIONAL STATISTICS
1994 - 1995

NORMAN M. BRADBURN (*Chair*), National Opinion Research Center, University of Chicago

JOHN E. ROLPH (*Vice Chair*), Department of Information and Operations Management, School of Business Administration, University of Southern California

JOHN F. GEWEKE, Department of Economics, University of Minnesota, Minneapolis

JOEL B. GREENHOUSE, Department of Statistics, Carnegie Mellon University

ERIC A. HANUSHEK, W. Allen Wallis Institute of Political Economy, Department of Economics, University of Rochester

ROBERT M. HAUSER, Department of Sociology and Institute for Research on Poverty, University of Wisconsin, Madison

NICHOLAS JEWELL, Vice Provost, Chancellor's Office, University of California, Berkeley

WILLIAM NORDHAUS, Department of Economics, Yale University

JANET L. NORWOOD, The Urban Institute, Washington, D.C.

EDWARD B. PERRIN, School of Public Health and Community Medicine, University of Washington

KEITH F. RUST, Westat, Inc., Rockville, Maryland

DANIEL L. SOLOMON, Associate Dean, Academic Affairs, North Carolina State University

MIRON L. STRAF, *Director*

Contents

Acknowledgments

The Board on Children and Families and the Committee on National Statistics wish to thank the authors of the papers in this volume, as well as the many presenters and discussants who provided thoughtful comments at the workshop. We especially thank Robert Hauser of the University of Wisconsin for serving as chair.

We also gratefully acknowledge the commitment and support of all those who worked collaboratively to organize the workshop and prepare this report. In the early stages of the project, Constance Citro, Deborah Phillips, and Miron Straf developed plans for the workshop. Nancy Maritato took the major responsibility for organizing the workshop and prepared an initial draft of the workshop summary. Drusilla Barnes and Agnes Gaskin assisted in the planning and organizing efforts. Deborah Phillips and Anne Bridgman took the lead in making revisions, responding to review, and preparing the final draft. Christine McShane edited the report and prepared it for publication.

Integrating Federal Statistics on Children

Interest in monitoring and understanding the lives of children has grown rapidly in recent years. Fueled in part by growing pressures to hold public programs accountable for outcomes, as well as by mounting concerns about the instability and apparently worsening problems that characterize the lives of many children, those who shape our nation's child policies are increasingly looking to the federal statistical system for answers to complex questions about the development of children in today's society. At the same time, the nation is contemplating a major shift in responsibility for several major children's programs from the federal to state governments. Such a shift will place even greater demands on the capacity of national data to track and release in a timely fashion information on the effects on children's well-being of this major redirection of public resources.

It is in this context that the Committee on National Statistics and the Board on Children and Families of the National Research Council and the Institute of Medicine convened a workshop to examine the adequacy of federal statistics on children and families. Through a series of background papers, discussants' remarks, and participant discussions, the workshop provided a forum for a preliminary assessment of the strengths and shortcomings of existing and proposed federal statistical data sources, particularly with respect to their capacity to fill the most pressing information needs of those who formulate, implement, and analyze policies for children.

The papers covered several types of data collection initiatives: (1) those designed to track the effects of major policy developments: we examined data needs related to health care reorganization (Newacheck and Starfield), but similar issues also pertain to policies in the area of public assistance and child welfare; (2) those designed primarily to explain the development and well-being of children, particularly across developmental transitions, such as school and work force entry, and with regard to the context of family, community, and government resources (Brooks-Gunn et al., Hofferth, Pallas); and (3) those designed to access the incidence, sequelae, and consequences of relatively rare but developmentally salient events, such as child abuse and other forms of violence involving children (Loftin and Mercy).

Over the course of the workshop, the discussion converged on several cross-cutting themes, and the participants made numerous suggestions—some highly detailed and others more general—for improving the existing statistical system. This introductory chapter highlights the common themes that emerged at the workshop, none of which should be viewed as formal consensus opinions, and concludes with a few ideas about next steps. The next chapter provides a summary of the workshop presentations and discussion. The five workshop papers conclude the body of the report.

CROSS-CUTTING THEMES

The title of the workshop itself reflects an assumption, amply confirmed by the participants, that federal statistical data on children and families are highly fragmented. Just as policy for children in the United States is best portrayed as an accumulation of responses to problems that are only rarely viewed as interrelated, federal statistics on children are far from being a coherent, logically developed system. Data collection efforts are highly fragmented, administered by different agencies, each with its own substantive interests and each with distinctive histories and constituencies. As noted in the paper by Aaron Pallas, this context must be taken into account in trying to understand why the "system" looks the way it does, and in attempting to address the key redundancies and gaps that characterize the existing collection of data resources. In effect, each of the participants grappled with the conclusion that we have both too many and too few statistical data on children.

Furthermore, the participants were cognizant of the limited, if not shrinking, funds for federal data collection efforts. The net effect of budgetary limitations on heightening pressures for greater efficiency and coordination across the federal statistical agencies and on constraining the range of possible responses to improving the existing system was a topic of substantial discussion at the workshop. With these shared concerns about fragmentation and resource constraints as a point of departure, the following common themes regarding problems and suggestions for improving federal statistics on children emerged from the workshop discussions.

- *Improvements in data are needed to understand the connections between resources and child outcomes, as well as the family and community processes that translate resources into outcomes.*

Many of the most pressing policy questions now center on identifying promising targets of intervention, whether the topic is preventing childhood illness, ensuring for children a successful start in school, or reducing inequitable patterns of school dropout and completion. Supplementing family income, changing parents' behavior through parent education or family planning interventions, investing in social services, and improving the neighborhoods and other settings in which children develop offer competing policy responses to a range of issues.

Answers to these questions emphasize the importance of collecting data that can be put to more than purely descriptive purposes. This, in turn, requires that careful assessment of resources and other inputs to children's development be accompanied by assessments of child outcomes *in the same survey*. Assessments of family functioning (e.g., communication patterns, supervision and discipline, the learning environment) and of the peer, schooling, and neighborhood-level settings and processes that can explain how resources affect outcomes would further enhance the capacity of childhood data to inform the efficient allocation of public resources toward the most potent sources of child well-being.

Although several major datasets (i.e., the Panel Study of Income Dynamics, the Survey of Income and Program Participation) provide relatively rich data on inputs to development and others focus on family functioning (i.e., the National Survey of Families and Households), data on child outcomes are substantially more limited, particularly during the pre-high-school years, and no single survey presently encompasses a good complement of measures of resources, processes, and outcomes. With respect to outcomes, the dearth of "positive" measures that will enable us to learn from those who fare well about the ingredients of successful development was specifically noted as a critical need to complement our current capacity to learn from those who fare poorly about the factors that compromise development.

Among the many types of resources that were discussed (e.g., monetary, psychological, human capital, community resources and networks, and resources that arise from government policies), the resource of parental time inputs surfaced as a major gap in current data collection efforts. Participants called for the addition of question sequences focused on parental time use to existing surveys, as well as for a separate national time use survey of children and their parents.

Beyond the simple accounting of resources, data collection on the organization and distribution of resources—notably health care, early education and schooling experiences—across subgroups of children was recommended.

This information is essential to assessing equity of access to public resources, as well as differential outcomes for children who might otherwise appear to grow up under similar circumstances. More careful measurement of income, including items that distinguish among various sources of income, capture what families do with their income, and assess the allocation of income (and other resources) across family members and continuing through the time when children move out of the parental home, was also highlighted as a major information need.

- *It is important to collect information on family relationships that goes beyond each member's relation to a single reference person, distinguishes among biological, step-, and adoptive parents, and includes noncustodial parents.*

Several presenters and discussants called attention to the value of establishing relations among all pairs of individuals in a household and of identifying the nature of the parent-child relationship (biological, stepparent, adoptive) for all child-parent dyads living in and out of the household. This is the only way in which relations among subgroups of family members, as well as issues that bear on differing degrees of genetic relatedness among caretakers and children, can be examined. Grandparent-child-grandchild relations, comparisons of developmental trajectories for siblings, and the role of noncustodial parents and nonresidential family members in children's lives were salient themes in the discussion. A related need concerned the inclusion of identifiers that enable the linkage of family members and the subsequent creation of family-level records in addition to individual and person records aimed at encouraging family-level data analysis of datasets ranging from the National Health Interview Survey to the Public Use MicroSample (PUMS) microdata files derived from the 1990 census.

Other presenters noted the limits of household-based surveys for addressing particular policy issues, notably those concerning violence against children and educational attainment and the transition to work. In the first case, exclusive reliance on a household-based sampling frame misses vital information on episodes of violence perpetrated by individuals who are weakly attached to the child's household. It also militates against important efforts to integrate information about child victimization at home, in school, and in other settings. In the second case, household surveys typically are not designed to ensure a sufficient sample of individuals within a particular organizational context, such as a school or workplace. These examples raise the methodological challenge of experimenting with unconventional sampling plans.

- *Given the current move toward block grants, the state and local locus of many policies and programs for children, and growing interest in the effects of state variation in benefit levels, service struc-*

tures, and other key features of social policy programs, there is a critical need for data that will allow for reliable state- and local-level estimates.

This recommendation surfaced with respect to every policy area discussed at the workshop. For example, health care reform is taking different forms in different states, yet none of the major federal health surveys has the capacity to assess the effects of state-level reform efforts on children and families. Pressing needs include the selection of primary sampling units that are consistent with state-level estimation, inclusion of a sufficient number of cases at the state level to permit accurate estimation, and making better use of claims data and other administrative records. The value of linking qualitative and local data to national health surveys in order to interpret local health care trends, processes, and effects on children and families was also noted. Similarly, efforts to track and prevent violence are implemented at the local level and require data that can produce small-area estimates. Presenters also called for adding state-of-residence identifiers to national data as a routine matter in order to encourage analysis of state-to-state variation in program benefits and structures.

The significant contribution to available information that would be made by appending neighborhood-based data to existing data files was also noted by several participants, particularly with respect to questions of local resources, economic opportunities, aggregate poverty levels, and other features of the surrounding population. Suggestions for enhancing capacity at state and local levels to conduct surveys and to collect useful administrative data were also made.

The broader issue in which this discussion was embedded concerned the importance of being able to link data across geographic levels (federal, state, local) for the purpose of examining the effects of how policies developed at different levels of government interact with each other and, in turn, create differing patterns of intended or unintended consequences for children. Coordination of data across other levels of analysis unique to particular issues was also discussed. Understanding the effects of health care reforms requires outcome data that can be aggregated at the patient-provider, plan or system of care, and community or population levels. Explanatory variables in datasets aimed at clarifying child development would ideally be measured at the household, community, institutional (i.e., schools), and state levels.

- *The changing demographics of the childhood population, as well as shifting policy concerns, require new strategies for oversampling currently under- and unrepresented subgroups of children.*

Each of the presenters noted that the most significant effects of policy developments are often experienced by groups of children that are seriously underrepresented or excluded from federal statistical data on children. Furthermore, rapid growth in immigrant families and the fact that many children experience shifting family structures call for a reassessment of the sampling strategies that are typically employed in federally supported surveys. Populations of particular concern vary somewhat by substantive area. For example, chronically ill children were identified as a critical subgroup to capture in health surveys; youth in prisons or jails, in the military, and those who were early school dropouts were identified with respect to surveys of the transition from school to work; and children of non-English-speaking parents were identified as a critical subgroup when studying the preschool and early school years.

Common across topics were calls to sample sufficient numbers of Hispanic and Asian children (and to disaggregate these broad categories into distinct subgroups, such as Mexican-Americans and Puerto Ricans), institutionalized and homeless children, children in out-of-home placements, and children with disabilities and other special needs. In light of immigration trends, calls were also made for routinely including information about length of time in the United States and country of origin for all family members.

- *Improved longitudinal data on children and families would facilitate efforts to address several critical policy issues pertaining to changes in family resources, predictors of successful development across key transition points, and the identification of early precursors of serious problems in middle childhood and adolescence.*

Among the pressing questions that require longitudinal data are: (1) How do changes in resources and family arrangements affect children? (2) What factors predict successful transitions into school and from schooling to work? (3) What are the long-term consequences of assaultive violence on children? (4) What is known about the sequencing of health events, as well as behavioral problems, over the course of development? It was uniformly perceived that available data are seriously inadequate to address these questions.

Numerous longitudinal surveys—both active and planned (e.g., the National Longitudinal Survey of Youth and its Child-Mother Supplement, the Survey of Income and Program Participation, the National Survey of Family Growth, the Early Childhood Longitudinal Survey)—were discussed. As a collection, however, they were portrayed as flawed by a wide range of problems. These include limited and unrepresentative target populations; problems with length (age range followed) and periodicity of data collection; specialized foci that militate against efforts to examine how behavior in one domain (i.e., health) interrelates with behavior in another domain (i.e., achievement); a failure to follow children across critical transition points, such as from the preschool to the school years; and sampling strategies that follow households or adults and therefore lose children as they shift from one household to another or move out of a family setting.

Although cognizant of the vast expense of mounting a new panel study of children and families—whether initiated with a new, independently sampled cohort of children or by augmenting an existing survey—several of the presenters felt that, if substantial new resources were devoted to federal statistics on children, this would be the wisest option to pursue. Other presenters noted that no single survey would ever address all of the information needs of policy makers and researchers and favored a more diversified approach. Each of the presenters and discussants made suggestions for lower-cost supplements to samples and items as well as other changes to existing surveys as a short-term strategy and one that would complement the longer-term strategy of developing a new national survey of children.

- *The critical need for improved cross-agency planning and coordination, as well as coordination across private and public data sources, emerged as a priority across the topical issues under discussion.*

As federal statistical data on children have accumulated, the databases from which these data derive have become increasingly specialized and categorical in nature. Furthermore, even within agencies, supplements, topical modules, and new surveys tend to proliferate with minimal attention to opportunities for linkages with existing data collection efforts. In the area of health care, the need to integrate data across public and private data collection organizations was noted as an additional challenge facing those who seek useful data about the course and effects of health care reforms.

The urgency of developing a cross-agency data coordinating mechanism that can direct efforts to reduce redundancies, cover gaps, standardize definitions and item formats, and, in general, establish a more efficient system, is compounded by current fiscal pressures. Furthermore, absent coordination, opportunities to share protocols and instruments, to consider complementary sampling strategies, to develop compatible data coding systems, and to collaborate on analyses and reporting of results will be missed. Calls were also made for a coordinated methodological research program aimed at such issues as techniques for improving the validity of responses to sensitive questions, controversial tensions that surround the need to protect respondent confidentiality, methods of linking data across surveys, and innovative approaches to collecting data from multiple informants and in new settings.

The model of the Federal Interagency Forum on Aging-Related Statistics, which was established to encourage cooperation among federal agencies in the development, collection, analysis, and dissemination of data on the older population, was noted as an effective mechanism for interagency communication. A promising development, since the workshop, is the formation of a Federal Interagency Forum on Child and Family Statistics. The forum, which is a voluntary mechanism to improve coordination of child and family data on behalf of the federal statistical agencies, offers the opportunity to engage in precisely the types of cross-agency planning suggested by the workshop participants.

NEXT STEPS

Over the course of the workshop, an ambitious set of suggestions for improving existing data and developing new data was made. Initial steps toward ensuring thoughtful and ongoing deliberations about the issues raised at the workshop were also suggested. These included:

- *Promoting collaborative meetings.* Participants noted an immediate opportunity to convene key federal statistical and research agencies (e.g., the National Institute on Mental Health, the National Institute on Child Health and Human Development, the Department of Education, the Department of Health and Human Services, the Bureau of the Census, the National Institute of Justice) for the purpose of sharing notes about surveys currently being planned. Along these lines, the value of developing an integrated consortium of sampling frames and topical modules for new surveys was noted.
- *Coordinating efforts aimed at supplementing existing datasets.* Numerous detailed suggestions were made by the workshop participants for improving the utility and quality of existing datasets. A forum for continuing this type of discussion and effective mechanisms for implementing agreed-on recommendations were viewed as pressing needs. Such a forum could also provide for consideration of the pros and cons of launching a new national survey of children.
- *Continuing to examine the fit between the information needs of decision makers and the terrain of available data.* A sustained debate among data developers and data users, including policy makers, centered on the degree to which available data match information needs, was viewed as a very promising avenue for guiding the future of the federal statistical system. Key players would include staff from the statistical agencies, academics, contractors, and policy experts from a variety of vantage points.
- *Addressing the underutilization of existing data.* Efforts to develop and disseminate means of encouraging greater access to existing data on behalf of evaluators and researchers not involved in the original data design and collection were also identified as warranting immediate attention. Specific suggestions included involving data users early on in the development of new surveys, ascertaining effective approaches to training new users, and developing more accessible, user-friendly data files.

Workshop Summary

The Committee on National Statistics and the Board on Children and Families of the National Research Council and the Institute of Medicine held a workshop on March 31 and April 1, 1994, to examine the adequacy of federal statistics on children and families. Concurrent with increased interest in monitoring and understanding the lives of children and families is a recognition of serious shortcomings in federal and other major longitudinal data used by policy makers to inform their work. Workshop participants, including staff of the statistical agencies that design and implement surveys, researchers who analyze statistical data, and policy experts who make use of these data to address pressing issues affecting children and families, discussed the following issues:

- What are the most pressing information needs of those who formulate, implement, and analyze policies for children and families?
- What are the strengths and shortcomings of existing and proposed federal statistical data sources for addressing these information needs? To what extent do existing sampling strategies follow children across critical transition points? Are there populations of children, such as immigrant children, for whom adequate data do not exist? To what extent is it possible to combine data to examine relations across domains of development, such as school achievement, health, and criminal behavior?
- What are the most promising strategies for improving the capacity of the federal statistical system to address these needs? Should the focus be

on enhancing the integration of existing data sets or developing a national survey of children?

Over the course of the workshop, participants considered these issues against the framework of key developmental transition points in children's lives from birth through preparation for adulthood. Using the presentations by the authors of five background papers as a basis, the participants discussed: (1) child development in the context of family and community resources; (2) children's transitions into school; (3) federal data on educational attainment and the transition to work; (4) the data needs for monitoring health care reform for children and families; and (5) estimating the incidence, causes, and consequences of interpersonal violence for children and families.

CHILD DEVELOPMENT IN THE CONTEXT OF FAMILY AND COMMUNITY RESOURCES

Jeanne Brooks-Gunn, Brett Brown, Greg Duncan, and Kristin Moore addressed the issue of improving national data to facilitate policy making for children and youth. Datasets must have reliable and, if possible, longitudinal assessments of child outcomes and measures should be age- and development-specific, the authors note. Sets of child supplements offer one approach to capturing such information. Assessments should cover as many of the crucial domains of child and adolescent development as possible, given a limited interview period. It may be best to link the timing of assessments to what is known regarding time frames of stability and change, e.g., family income.

Since resources, broadly conceived, are instrumental in promoting or retarding development, a high-quality, longitudinal measurement of family income, by source of income as well as amount, is crucial for testing resource-based theories of child and adolescent development, the authors note. In addition, time resources, especially parents' time spent with children, are typically neglected or not measured well, although they are crucial resources. Measures of other family process mediators are needed to understand the ways in which resources affect child development. Datasets should include information from as many sources as possible, since resources can come from the neighborhood, the school, and the community, as well as the family. In addition to resources, it is important that data collection allows for the development of dynamic measures of family structure, especially since the changing structure of American families is likely to have a large impact on children and adolescents.

The list of additions proposed by the authors to the many national data collection projects reviewed is long and expensive, and funds are probably insufficient to support all of these augmentations and also fund a new national survey of children. Therefore, it is important to consider whether it would be better to allocate resources in a piecemeal fashion across existing surveys or to attempt to pool those resources and spend a substantial fraction of them on a new panel study focused exclusively on child and adolescent development.

No-cost and low-cost additions to existing surveys should be top priorities, the authors note. However, in considering the trade-offs between recommending high-cost additions to existing surveys and the fielding of a new survey, a new survey may be the best use of available resources because, although many of the existing datasets provide valuable information on child development, they were either designed for other purposes or are designed too narrowly to serve as a general resource for research on children.

Discussant Gary Sandefur commented that investment in a new longitudinal survey of children would be useful in estimating causal models of child development, but it would not fully identify the most pressing information needs of those who formulate, implement, and analyze policies for children and families. For those using data in policy development, especially those who cannot wait for a new survey, Sandefur called for a focus on such predictor variables as income, family functioning, community resources, and instability.

Data users need better measurements of what families are doing with their income—how it is utilized and how it affects such child outcomes as high school graduation and teenage pregnancy, he suggested. It is also important to consider what income provides access to, including material resources, opportunities, and perceived security. Family functions, such as time use and how it changes and parent practices in terms of supervision and discipline, are also important, as are the characteristics and availability of community resources and differing patterns of utilization of these resources by children and families. Instability, in resources and in where and with whom children live, must also be captured by major data collection efforts. These underlying variables, as well as changes over time, are possible causes of child outcomes, such as health, educational attainment, and employment.

A tension exists between short-run scientific and policy needs and long-term needs. Proposals for new surveys would, in the long run, meet the information needs identified, as well as make possible broader and richer policy and scientific research. But quickly addressing gaps in our knowledge could be done in the context of existing studies, such as the National Longitudinal Survey of Youth Child-Mother Supplement and the Survey of Income and Program Participation (SIPP) Child Module, Sandefur noted. Given limited national resources for data collection, the choice between a new survey and supplementation of existing surveys is difficult to make; indeed, they are most appropriately viewed as complementary strategies.

Discussant Donald Hernandez responded to several suggestions in the Brooks-Gunn et al. paper by explaining current and proposed changes in data collection by the Census Bureau:

- The Census Bureau is planning a Survey of Program Dynamics (SPD), which will follow the entire 1993 SIPP panel for an additional seven years, much of it devoted to measuring child well-being.
- The 1996 SIPP panel will identify each parent of a child who lives in the household; this approach will be extended in order to identify biological, step-, and adoptive parent-child relationships.
- The 1990 decennial census effort to explicitly identify biological and stepchildren met with limited success; unless a new approach to data collection is developed, a strong case for the uses of these data would be required.
- Likewise, very strong cases would be required in order for the Census Bureau to consider restoring the marital history question and identify children who are in school.
- Speaking to suggestions that the Census Bureau consider producing a matched file with family and neighborhood-level data from the 1990 census comparable to similar files produced from the 1970 and 1980 census, Hernandez commented that, if the demand for such data were documented and a funding source identified, the Census Bureau would no doubt produce such a data file.
- The suggestion that the Census Bureau should consider creating family-level records in addition to household and person records for their PUMS microdata files is feasible, but the case needs to be made to justify the additional expenditures required.

Turning to SIPP, Hernandez noted that specific improvements suggested in the paper—data on child outcomes and on the family processes that translate resources into child outcomes and a broader array of resources, for example—are high on the list of important areas to be considered for inclusion. Responding to a criticism that SIPP has a relatively small sample size, limiting efforts to minimize attrition and to follow any children who leave the household, Hernandez said the sample size in the 1996 SIPP will be larger (about 34,000 children).

A proposed Survey of Child and Adolescent Development, suggested in the paper as an alternative to high-cost augmentations, warrants thorough evaluation, Hernandez said. He and the authors discussed the design and implementation of such a survey. Since the 1996 SIPP panel will be collecting much of the needed data on income, program participation, family change, etc., that will be essential for a national survey of child and adolescent development, Hernandez noted that it may be that the most cost-effective approach to fielding the survey will be to use the 1996 SIPP panel as the basic data collection vehicle.

The content of new questions and new surveys generated lively discussion among the workshop participants. Some agreed on the need for a well-informed, thoughtful process to inform hard choices about investing federal resources for data collection on children, including decisions regarding whether or not to support the costs of a new child-focused survey. Others, who thought it unwise to put all one's eggs in one basket, called for maintaining a variety of surveys. There was further discussion of the challenges of any effort to design and implement a new, comprehensive national survey on children, including the difficulty of pooling money across federal agencies and time constraints on data collection in homes. The content of new questions and new surveys generated discussion on genetic relatedness of family members, creative uses of sibling data, expanded indices of social and economic status, and time use.

A number of workshop participants cited the importance of being able to follow children longitudinally as they move from the households where information is originally obtained to other households and settings over the course of their development. The participants also discussed the value of using an integrated consortium of sampling frames (i.e., households, schools, health and service organizations) for a new survey in order to capture multiple perspectives on children's development.

CHILDREN'S TRANSITION TO SCHOOL

Sandra Hofferth outlined the scientific issues involved in evaluating children's transition to school. Developmental outcomes in this transitional period are typically categorized into three groups: the cognitive domain, including language and achievement; the socioemotional domain, including self-concept, social interaction, and behavioral problems; and the health domain, including physical development and abilities and good health habits. The national objectives in the Goals 2000 law add approaches to learning and language usage to the set of categories.

Children receive a number of inputs: not only do they receive financial contributions from parents, but they also receive valuable resources such as time, care, and attention from them. Development is also influenced by the environment in which children are raised, including the social and economic environment and the stability of these circumstances. Mediating factors during early childhood, such as parenting style, communication, attitudes, and beliefs, also affect later well-being. Moderating factors such as temperament, parent, family, community, neighborhood, and school characteristics are also important.

Research has demonstrated a relationship between early behavior problems and later problems in school and antisocial activities, implying that programs to reduce aggressive behavior should be developed in the early childhood years. However, the effectiveness of such activity has rarely been addressed. A cost-effectiveness analysis of different approaches would be beneficial. Since the only way to address the relevant questions is through scientific analyses that compare the relative effects of these different factors in one model, it is important that models be as comprehensive as possible, including all potential mediators to the extent possible.

Hofferth identified several evaluation studies that currently exist and four studies that will potentially fill some of the gaps. Some gaps, however, will remain, including the lack of a longitudinal study of a national representative sample of children starting prior to school entry and following children into school, lack of state-level measures, lack of collection of time-use data, and small sample sizes.

To fill the remaining gaps, Hofferth recommended supplementing ongoing collections, such as the Panel Study of Income Dynamics and the National Longitudinal Survey of Youth Child-Mother Supplement. A coordinated data collection effort providing some overlap between surveys would also improve the situation, since it would allow for more cross-study comparisons and validation than previously possible. Another approach would involve implementing new surveys, such as a national survey of children and a national time-use survey of children and their parents.

Discussant John Love addressed one of the central implicit questions of the workshop as it applies to children's transition into school: What statistics are required to design, implement, and evaluate policies aimed at improving the health and well-being of children and families? Love noted the importance of studying the transition into school, pointing out that the way in which this transition is handled could make a difference in extending the benefits of children's preschool experiences. If there are disruptive effects of discontinuity of experience as children enter school, understanding the nature of this transition can help minimize them.

Love expanded Hofferth's three basic scientific questions to account for disparities between age groups, address transition processes in and of themselves, and examine specific inputs that are related either to the transition event or the transition period. He also suggested several additional questions:

- What are the important transitions at the time of school entry? Cataloging these and learning more about how prevalent each is—how many children experience each type of transition—are prerequisites to deciding what policy questions are important to address with federal statistics.
- What differences do transitions make in children's lives? Currently,

we can only conjecture about how children's experiences of transitions affect their later school success.

- What is the period of transition into school? Evidence indicates that kindergarten serves as a transition from preschool to first grade. A full understanding of transitions at the time of school entry will not be possible until we develop ways of describing children's experience across this one-year period. But if we consider the school entry transition as a period of time rather than a point in time, this will affect the statistics that are needed, according to Love.

In order to sort out information priorities, a consensus effort is needed aimed at identifying the most important things to know about how well children are doing during this transition period and what inputs are most important to understand. Also, a reasonable number of specific transitions should be decided on; Love sees the transitions from home to school, from Head Start to school, and from child care to school as the most important. Finally, more should be learned to elucidate how the features of transition experiences make a difference in such areas as children's adjustment to kindergarten and in the dimensions of development that have been identified as important for school readiness.

Discussant Jerry West agreed with the need for a careful conceptualization of the transition from preschool to school in order to guide this area of federal statistics on children. A model should be developed that represents a long-term process from birth to the point of entry and to subsequent outcomes. Such a model would require the collection of information on a wide range of outcomes; careful assessments of children's experiences in classrooms and in the family would also be beneficial. Although there is a changing conceptualization of education and of what is important regarding understanding school performance, there is a paucity of data that allow us to look at this issue. In addition, data that will permit examination of links between inputs and outputs are needed.

West called for a new generation of studies that involve a collaborative effort between private and public agencies and between disciplines, preferably through a systematic approach and starting with a birth cohort. Data users should be involved early in the development of such a survey, he advised.

Workshop participants agreed that the absence of data following children from preschool into school constitutes a serious gap in the federal statistical system, particularly given the growth in reliance on child care and the debate over school readiness. In this context, they returned to several themes raised earlier during the workshop:

- The tension between starting anew with a survey of children and supplementing existing datasets,
- The difficulty of capturing the *process* of development using survey methods, and
- The challenges associated with integrating federal datasets given survey-specific constructs, definitions, and survey items.

Participants also stressed the importance of creating an effective mechanism for interagency communication about data collection, based perhaps on the Federal Forum on Aging.

EDUCATIONAL ATTAINMENT AND TRANSITION INTO WORK

Aaron Pallas examined institutionally based data that are designed to illuminate the role of schooling and the process of transition into the labor force. Many of the important analytic policy questions regarding the transition to work view the youth labor market in the context of its connections to other social institutions, such as schools, families, and communities. Thus, attention is directed to what might be called the school-to-work transition system, or the linkage system that joins school and the economy.

Among the key weaknesses in the available data sources that address education-to-work experiences are the kinds of questions asked. The failure to include measures of theoretically relevant constructs in attempts to model or understand complex social phenomena (such as efforts to measure cognitive ability) results in specification error. Also, the relevant theoretical constructs are sometimes measured poorly, resulting in measurement error. The second weakness involves the issue of when are questions asked. In periods of relatively rapid educational reform and economic change, it may be desirable to address questions about high school completion, postsecondary access and persistence, and youth labor market experience much more frequently than every 8 or 10 years, as is the current practice. A third weakness is that household surveys typically are not designed to ensure a critical mass or cluster of individuals within a particular organizational context, such as a school. Yet studies of individuals independent of the school and workplace contexts in which they are situated may not reveal the important role that schools and employers play in structuring educational attainment and the transition into the labor force.

To improve the capacity of the federal statistical system to address information needs, Pallas suggested:

- Conducting a needs assessment in order to understand the current data available and how well it meets the information needs of policy makers,

• Establishing an interagency working group, composed of the agencies that work with data that shed light on the well-being of children, to examine the gaps, overlaps, and redundancies in the current federal statistical system, and
• Establishing an oversight committee with the responsibility of arbitrating among different agency interests.

Pallas also cautioned that broad federal statistical data collections that function as systems are not a substitute for program evaluation. Targeted studies of particular programs and policies and specific target populations are a more fruitful source of information about how such programs and policies work.

Discussant Russell Rumberger acknowledged that a comprehensive and integrated statistical system is needed to understand and address the complex problems confronting American youth today. Although federal data collection efforts have recognized this need over time, there is still room for improvement.

Rumberger discussed four areas in which improvements can be made to provide better and more comprehensive information on children. The first improvement involves the type of questions asked. To understand and address the problems of children and youth, it is important to obtain simultaneous information about the characteristics and conditions of the children themselves as well as the characteristics and conditions of the settings in which they live, work, and go to school. Little is known about community and work settings and how they interact with children's home environments, even though experiences in those settings and interactions among them can significantly influence cognitive and social development.

Another improvement involves information on processes. A number of domains shape the development of children, including the cognitive, psychosocial, and health domains, as revealed in their knowledge and skills, attitudes and values, behaviors, and status. Typically much more information is collected on status variables (i.e., scores on achievement tests) than on process variables (i.e., whether children know how to acquire new information to inform new questions). Although enrollment and dropout status are commonly measured, for example, these status measures are necessarily arbitrary and reveal very little about the extent to which students are actually engaged in the schooling process and learning.

The collection of more longitudinal data rather than cross-sectional data would also be useful. In addition, more information should be collected on high-risk or vulnerable populations, such as institutional or minority groups, that are often undersampled or completely ignored in major federal data collection efforts.

Rumberger also called for better use of administrative records, more multimethod studies, more geographic detail, and use of common definitions and unique identifiers. He also suggested that more attention be paid to the use of federal data, rather than simply the generation of it. An information "cross-walk" could serve to index all current data available across agencies on related topics.

Discussant Suzanne Bianchi pointed out that, given the trends of increased inequality of earnings by educational attainment, restructuring of manufacturing, and the downsizing that seems to be affecting white-collar workers, the interrelationship of schooling and work is of increased importance to the well-being of not only the individuals involved, but also the dependents their work supports, especially dependent children. Current data collection efforts should adequately analyze this phenomenon.

In order to study adequately the transition from school to work and the connectedness of learning in school and performing on the job, it would be best to capture the student in school (taking into account aspects of the school context) and follow him or her to a job (taking into account work setting). Broad-based household surveys do not allow researchers to understand the aspects of schools that help or hinder new labor force entrants' productivity on the job or how work settings utilize, add to, and detract from the cognitive abilities and training that workers bring to the labor market. Most analysis begins with an implicit assumption that schooling translates into productivity in the labor market; however, this is a hypothesis that should be fully investigated by those studying the school-to-work transition.

Although the lack of data on individuals embedded in organizational settings is a limitation, the underutilization of existing data, particularly longitudinal data from the National Center for Education Statistics (NCES), is also a problem. Such data may shed light on school-to-work transition. NCES data could be improved by shortening the 10-year gap that separates longitudinal cohorts to allow for some short-term 2- to 3-year studies. Bianchi also noted the potential of SIPP to address school-to-work transitions. A pairing of the Census Bureau with NCES could help in carrying out this work, she said, though she noted that team approaches are costly and hard to execute.

Workshop participants touched on the importance of considering sampling frames and approaches that extend beyond the household unit and of obtaining data from multiple informants (e.g., employee and employer, students, teachers, and school administrators). They also addressed the need to standardize measures of educational status across surveys. Participants deplored the dearth of information about unconventional forms of employment, including underground employment, and the related lack of information regarding paths to conventional work choices.

MONITORING CHANGES IN HEALTH CARE FOR CHILDREN AND FAMILIES

In order to monitor significant changes in health care for children and families, information is needed to evaluate the state of health of the population, the adequacy of access to health care services, and the equity of use of services across different groups of individuals, according to authors Paul Newacheck and Barbara Starfield. Other pressing data needs include: information on how services are targeted to the needs of the population served; the extent to which services are accessible, comprehensive, and coordinated; and the extent to which provided services are justified by evidence of effectiveness and appropriateness. Policy makers also need information about the organization and distribution of resources within the health care system.

Newacheck and Starfield listed the five types of sources that are currently available for obtaining such information—vital statistics and surveillance systems, population surveys, provider surveys, administrative records, and health systems data—noting that only a few of the existing databases contain data across the multiple domains relevant to health care. As a result, they suggested, it may be desirable to integrate data at several levels. Linking data can yield significant benefits but presents additional challenges, including the need for clarity in concept development, standardization of measurement, assignment of personal identifiers that maintain confidentiality, and accountability mechanisms.

Given that limited funds are likely to be available for the monitoring system, the authors see a need for analysis of the marginal costs and marginal benefits of adding components to existing or newly developed monitoring systems. As much as possible, the system should rely on existing databases, modifying them as needed while keeping in mind their original purposes.

Discussant Nicholas Zill pointed to the rapid pace of health care reorganization and the important role assigned to health care data as a source of quality monitoring as critical contexts for considering future data needs in this area. In light of budgetary constraints, Zill called for a clear-eyed look at what is vital in current systems and what is expendable and could, as a result, provide opportunities for reallocating funding for more useful data collection. Although there is usefulness in preserving certain elements of the current health care data system, it is also important to recognize the changing health care needs of children (e.g., health problems that arise from social circumstances, such as exposure to violence) and the lack of data to inform decision makers about whether *these* needs are being met.

Zill noted that the Early Childhood Longitudinal Survey, the State and Local Area Immunization Coverage and Health Survey, and the SIPP Child

Module are under way. However, in part because different agencies are funding different pieces, they are proceeding without coordination.

Additional data are needed about patient-provider relationships, health plans, and local communities and populations in order to draw an accurate picture of how health care reorganization affects children and families, according to discussant Robert Valdez. Valdez commented that many of the surveys that can be used to address health care issues are inadequate to the task of monitoring health care reform; they should be complemented with qualitative and local data that can be used to interpret local health care trends, processes, and effects on children and families.

In a discussion of this issue, workshop participants cited the critical need for cross-agency planning and coordination in monitoring health care, from the development of common constructs (i.e., concepts of children's health status) to standardized questions and response choices across surveys. They also touched on the tensions surrounding the establishment of unique identifiers in health care data, notably the value of identifiers for data integration that stands alongside concerns about confidentiality. Participants talked about the importance of carefully considering the appropriate sampling frame (i.e., local, state, national) when collecting health data for various purposes. Several participants commented on the challenges associated with including subgroups of children that are often neglected in national data collection efforts, including institutionalized children and those in multicustody arrangements.

INTERPERSONAL VIOLENCE INVOLVING CHILDREN AND FAMILIES

The definition of violence as any use of force or threat of force, regardless of intent or magnitude, raises fundamental questions regarding the nature of interpersonal violence and the difficulties involved in measuring it. Colin Loftin and James Mercy addressed data collection activities that bear on serious assaultive violence in primary relationships, such as families, and violence involving children.

Three household surveys and four organization-based surveys are currently used to collect data on serious interpersonal assaultive violence. Among the pressing needs in the area of information about violence are the development of improved methods for eliciting valid responses about complex, sensitive, and traumatic violent incidents. It is often difficult to obtain information on violence to children, especially because the abuser is often present in the setting in which the interview is conducted. There must also be improved coverage of persons who are marginally attached to households, and methodological research on coverage must be undertaken. More information is needed about risk factors, social context, consequences, and sequences of violent episodes. Also, more and better information is needed about precursors and long-term consequences of severe assaultive violence. Finally, estimates of the incidence of serious assaultive violence in state and local areas are needed.

Loftin and Mercy called for a coordinated federal focus on data related to violence within and across agencies. They also recommended a coordinated methodological research program on issues that cut across data systems; the exploration of more efficient ways to identify cases; and an exploration of the feasibility of collecting data on violence in key heath care settings—and the training of health care providers to recognize cases.

Discussant David Cantor noted that surveys offer several important advantages as a source of information. Surveys can fill in the gaps left by administrative systems. For example, the police collect information only on the incidents that are reported to them, which, at best, constitute only 70 to 75 percent of all crimes; crimes are even less well reported by youths ages 12 to 19. In addition, surveys help ensure centralization of quality as well as standardization, whereas administrative records are subject to unknown quality controls and decentralized data collection. Finally, surveys are consistent in their use of terms, although there is not necessarily uniform adherence to definitions at the administrative level, especially across local and state jurisdictions.

Cantor noted, however, that surveys also have disadvantages involving the validity of measures of violence as reported by either victims or offenders and including the confidentiality/sensitivity of information provided, errors in survey design, and coverage problems.

The Child Abuse Prevention, Adoption, and Family Services Act of 1988 created an interagency Task Force on Child Abuse and Neglect, as noted by discussant Michael Rand. However, estimating the incidence, causes, and consequences of interpersonal violence of children and families involves more than better cooperation or improved coordination. Child maltreatment encompasses not only physical abuse, but also psychological abuse, neglect, and sexual abuse; the agencies that handle each of these problems work from different perspectives. Their different missions and perspectives result in different data needs, emphases, and even definitions of basic constructs. Differences and conflicts need to be identified and resolved if agencies with different mandates and perspectives are to coordinate efforts to improve estimates of the incidence and prevalence of the problem, he suggested.

There is a clear need to improve the ability to quantify child abuse and neglect. Although partial information is available through several sources, efforts to develop a composite are difficult; one major problem is that the definition of what constitutes child abuse is not agreed on. In addition, abuse occurs in a range of settings, and no database currently assesses incidence across settings.

A broad approach to data collection is one possible solution to the problem of differential definitions, needs, and perspectives, Rand posited. Information could be collected on all forms of violence and abusive behavior, and those deemed not sufficiently serious or not of specific interest to the agency could be discarded. However this approach may not solve all of the problems of a lack of consensus given that any data collection effort is necessarily constrainted by the underlying definitions and principles that guide it. Furthermore, definitional inconsistencies are not the only problem of measuring child abuse; because of the private nature of most violent acts, many subjects—especially children—are very sensitive to providing any information about the incident.

Rand agreed with Loftin and Mercy that federal agencies with interests in child and family violence and abuse should coordinate efforts to design an improved mechanism to produce statistics on child and family violence. The interagency Task Force on Child Abuse and Neglect can be an integral part of such a coordination effort. Rand suggested that, although efforts to coordinate federal child abuse statistics may be extremely difficult given the different perspectives and objectives of each of the federal agencies involved, the potential benefits of cooperative efforts make it imperative to undertake the effort.

In the discussion, workshop participants noted that a great deal of research is exploring more effective data collection methods in the area of interpersonal violence. For example, the National Institute of Justice is experimenting with questions that tap personal perceptions of safety. A youth risk supplement has been added to the National Health Interview Survey, using a portable tape recorder and a personal computer to ensure respondents' confidentiality (technology that is being considered for the National Crime Survey). In this case, respondents do not give their responses to the interviewer, but rather enter them directly as anonymous data. The child supplement to the Health Interview Survey may also add questions on discipline practices, which some feel step over the line between nonviolent and violent behavior. Participants cited additional problems confronting data collection on violence:

- Definitions of neglect vary by state, making it difficult to understand, let alone integrate, the information that is collected on this topic.
- Although the co-occurrence of child abuse and domestic violence in the same households is a pressing policy concern, no datasets currently exist that allow for the examination of this issue.
- Similarly, data do not exist to allow for integrating information about child victimization at home, in school, and in other settings.

- Institutional review boards can provide barriers to collecting data on violent behavior.
- Although violence has been identified as a major public health problem, it is not clear if data collection efforts in the context of health care reform will include this type of outcome.

Workshop Papers

Child Development in the Context of Family and Community Resources: An Agenda for National Data Collections

Jeanne Brooks-Gunn, Brett Brown, Greg J. Duncan, and Kristin Anderson Moore

INTRODUCTION

The last decade has witnessed a remarkable transformation in social science data and research on child and adolescent development. Coming from quite different starting points, child development researchers, sociologists, and economists have converged in their needs for rich, multilevel data based on large samples. Beginning from an interest in socioeconomic attainment, sociologists and economists have produced a burgeoning literature on the factors that foster and undermine attainment; they now find themselves needing to delve deeper into the processes labeled *socioeconomic status* to understand how individual characteristics and family processes interact with community influences to produce socioeconomic attainment. Developmentalists have a tradition of conducting rich and detailed studies using small samples to examine in depth the processes by which children's characteristics interact with parental socialization practices during childhood. This approach has produced a voluminous literature that now seeks to test its theories and findings with data based on larger, more representative samples. This intersection of interests from the fields of

Jeanne Brooks-Gunn is at the Center for the Study of Children and Families, Teachers College, Columbia University. Brett Brown and Kristin Anderson Moore are at Child Trends, Inc., Washington, D.C. Greg J. Duncan is at the Center for Urban Affairs and Policy Research, Northwestern University.

child development, sociology, and economics places great demands on existing data systems (Brooks-Gunn et al., 1991; Duncan, 1991; Cherlin, 1991).

Despite an almost exclusive concentration on problem behaviors and a paucity of theoretical models that evaluate the full set of factors that influence children's development (Bronfenbrenner, 1979), the evolving literature is demonstrating that individual, family, neighborhood, and school variables all contribute to children's development (Brooks-Gunn et al., 1993a; Rosenbaum and Popkin, 1991; Alexander et al., 1993; Furstinberg et al., 1987; Rutter, 1985; Maccoby and Martin, 1983; Eccles, 1983; Sigel, 1985; Werner and Smith, 1982; Moore et al., 1994; Duncan et al., 1994a). However, findings on the relative importance of these domains in determining varied outcomes await both better data and further research.

Common to most of this research is the predominant use of large national datasets compiled by federal agencies or by survey organizations funded by federal agencies. Some of these datasets, such as High School and Beyond and the National Educational Longitudinal Surveys, were designed explicitly by the National Center for Educational Statistics (NCES) for analyses of adolescent outcomes and transitions to adulthood. Others, such as the Child Supplements to the National Longitudinal Surveys of Youth, are based on question modules added to datasets conceived primarily for other (in this case, labor market) purposes. Researchers working with still other datasets, such as decennial census microdata files with matched family- and neighborhood-level data, have been able to conduct valuable research on adolescent behavior by exploiting existing information that has been organized into a more useful form.

Stimulated by the increasingly widespread and complex nature of social problems involving children and adolescents (National Commission on Children, 1991; Hernandez, 1993), federal efforts to initiate or supplement data collection activities appear to be increasing. This is reflected in plans in the Survey of Income and Program Participation for a new supplemental module on family processes and developmental outcomes, NCES's initiation of a large cohort study of 5-year-olds, and consideration by the National Center for Health Statistics of a 1996 Child and Family Health Survey as part of the National Health Interview Survey.

In this paper we suggest specific national data collection projects that could improve research on child and adolescent development.[1] Our explicit aim is to encourage continued expansion of both the outcome domains covered and the explanatory variables measured, to enhance the richness and quality of the data obtained, and to improve the representativeness of the samples that are drawn. These improvements would serve both the policy and academic research communities in their efforts to specify and estimate causal models of child, adolescent, and young adult behavior.

To this end, we begin with developmental theory and summarize key elements of an emerging "resource" framework, which we believe provides an integrative framework for understanding how child and adolescent development is affected by the time, money, and emotional resources of parents; by the institutions and "social capital" present in communities and neighborhoods; and by government policies that shape the context within which parental choices are made.

Next we explain and provide empirical examples of key elements of datasets that have proved especially useful in testing and drawing policy conclusions from the theoretical framework we advocate. Some of the elements we list consist of the outcomes, resources, and family processes identified by theory as important. Others are important methods for implementing and estimating child development models. Many of the illustrations are based on results from smaller-scale studies; all have implications for the data collection improvements we outline in this paper.

As we detail in the sections that follow, when assessing outcomes, a number of features are critical:

- *High-quality, longitudinal assessments of child outcomes,* obtained from the child as well as the parent and, when necessary, by trained professionals who test the child directly, and assessing how the factors that affect children influence development over periods of a decade or more;
- *Measurement of age-appropriate outcomes and transitions*; and
- *Outcomes measured across multiple domains of functioning.*

Also, as we discuss, measurement of resources needs to attend to the following:

- *High-quality, longitudinal measurement of family resources*, that is, obtaining measures of a broad range of economic and social resources periodically over the years when a child or adolescent is growing up;
- *Measures of time "inputs,"* including the amount of time, the activities engaged in, and the persons present and interacting with a child;
- *Measurement of family-process mediators*, such as communication patterns, disciplinary style, and teaching style;
- *Multiple levels of measurement*, including the child, the family, the school, the community, the neighborhood, and the state;
- *Measurement of school conditions*, such as school organization and the socioeconomic composition of the school;
- *Exact measurement of intrafamily relationships*; and
- *Measurement of extended-family relationships*, including relationships with grandparents, aunts, and uncles.

Methodological and sampling considerations are also important, including:

- *"Natural experiment" methods of model testing;*
- *Leverage for policy analyses provided by state-to-state variation* in program benefits and structure;
- *Oversamples of minority groups;*
- *Multiple informants*; and
- *Procedures to minimize and adjust for attrition in longitudinal surveys.*

We next review the content of 12 existing national data collections in light of our list of desirable design features of developmental modeling, including:

(1) Consumer Expenditure Surveys;
(2) Decennial census;
(3) High School and Beyond;
(4) National Crime Victimization Survey;
(5) National Educational Longitudinal Survey of 1988;
(6) National Health Interview Survey (NHIS) — Child Health Supplement 1988;
(7) National Longitudinal Survey of Youth (1979 Cohort);
(8) NLSY Child-Mother Data;
(9) National Survey of Families and Households;
(10) Panel Study of Income Dynamics;
(11) National Survey of Children; and
(12) Survey of Income and Program Participation.

Table 1 lists salient characteristics of each survey, including measures of family resources and processes, measures of the extrafamilial context (e.g., neighborhood, school, peer group, county, and state), special advantages and disadvantages, sample size, and periodicity. Table 2 summarizes available child outcome measures for each survey by age group.

Our theoretical discussion and empirical illustrations lead us directly to a set of suggested improvements, involving both incremental and more substantial investments in federal datasets that would enhance their value for research on child and adolescent development. In some cases, the suggestions involve minor and quite inexpensive changes that would produce large analytic benefits. In others, more expensive changes could open up invaluable analytic opportunities. We conclude with ideas for an even more expensive undertaking, a new longitudinal survey of children, outlining key design elements of such a survey.

FAMILY AND COMMUNITY RESOURCES AND CHILDREN'S DEVELOPMENT OVER TIME

Many different frameworks have been used to study how children develop and the factors that influence development during childhood, adolescence, and the early stages of adult life. Such frameworks include: family systems approaches, risk and resilience, family and extra-family ecology, the life course, and economic decision making. Almost all of them consider, at least in passing, the ecology in which development occurs (context), as well as the stage or phase of life in which an individual is placed (time). However, these frameworks differ markedly in their relative emphases on time and context. Moreover, they also differ in how they examine the individual moving through time and context. Increasing interest in interdisciplinary research has focused attention on the value of different frameworks as well as the importance of looking at multiple mechanisms underlying development in any one study (Brooks-Gunn, in press; Brooks-Gunn et al., 1991; Duncan, 1991; Cherlin, 1991).

A number of investigative teams now combine scholars of macro issues (economists, sociologists, and demographers) and scholars concerned with more micro-oriented issues (developmental and clinical psychologists, pediatricians). Examples of such endeavors include Cherlin et al. (1991), Duncan et al. (1994a), Baydar and Brooks-Gunn (1991), Baydar et al. (1993), and Desai et al. (1989). The National Institute of Child Health and Human Development (NICHD) has recently initiated a Family and Child Well-Being Research Network, comprised of seven researchers and their colleagues; the seven teams in the NICHD network represent all six disciplines mentioned above.

Discipline-focused perspectives can be integrated into a framework based on familial and extrafamilial resources. The model we employ borrows heavily from the work of Coleman on social capital theory (1988) as well as the recent work by Haveman and Wolfe on choice-investment theory (1994). However, it departs from these two efforts in making more explicit the links with disciplines that focus on familial and extrafamilial processes, e.g., systems theory, ecological theory, and psychological-resource or social-support theory.

Resources

Like Haveman and Wolfe (1994), we view "resources" very broadly, defining them as consisting of the money, time, interpersonal connections, and institutions that parents and communities may use to promote the development of children. Resources actually spent on promoting child and adolescent development are considered "investments" since, independent of

TABLE 1 Review of Federal Survey Contents and Characteristics

Survey	Family Material Resources	Family Process	Contextual Data
Panel Study of Income Dynamics (PSID)	income source welfare hlthins assets tenure month year multi	spend marhist biopar	neighhd zip county state move
National Longitudinal Survey of Youth (NLSY)	income source welfare hlthins assets tenure month year	time biopar	school county state peer move
National Longitudinal Survey of Youth—Child-Mother Data (NLSY-CM)	income source welfare hlthins assets tenure month year	ppcnflct commun marhist biopar	county state move
National Educational Longitudinal Survey of 1988 (NELS88)	income assets multi	time activty rules commun spend	neighhd school
National Survey of Children (NSC)	income source welfare tenure multi	time activty ppcnflct pccnflct soccap rules commun violnce marhist deprsn biopar	neighhd school zip state peers move

Survey Characteristics

Special Advantages	Special Problems	Sample Size	Periodicity
sibs black Latino absparent exact tract	foster institut	4,800 households in 1968; 7,900 households in 1993	Annual, since 1968
sibs black Latino child exact cheval	nopar	12,686 in 1979	Annual, since 1979
sibs black Latino exact cheval	follow foster institut unrep	6,503 children in 1992	1986, 88, 90, 92, 94, (biennial)
Latino Asian child teach exact	foster	24,599 in 1988; 21,188 in 1992	1988, 90, 92, 94, 98
sibs black child abspar teach exact cheval	institut	2,301 in 1976; 1,147 in 1987	1976, 1981, 1987

TABLE 1 Continued

Survey	Family Material Resources	Family Process	Contextual Data
Survey of Income and Program Participation (SIPP)	income source welfare hlthins assets	marhist biopar	state move
National Survey of Families and Households (NSFH)	income source welfare assets tenure multi	time activty ppcnflct pccnflct soccap rules commun violnce marhist deprsn biopar	county move
High School and Beyond (HS&B)	income source welfare assets tenure multi	commun spend	school peer
Consumer Expenditure Surveys (CEX)	income source welfare hlthins assets tenure	spend	
National Crime Victimization Survey (NCVS)	income hlthins tenure year	violnce	move
Decennial Census, Public Use Micro-Sample (5%)	income source welfare tenure		county state move

Survey Characteristics

Special Advantages	Special Problems	Sample Size	Periodicity
bothpar absparent exact sibs	follow institut	20,000 households in 1993	Every 4 months for 30 months
sib black Latino child bothpar absparent exact	institut	13,017 households in 1987-1988; 7,926 children	1987-1988, 1992-1993
sib black Latino teach cheval	foster nopar	58,270 in 1980; 24,354 in 1986	1980, 82, 84 86; 1992 (small sub-sample)
	foster institut	5,000 households	Every quarter for 5 quarters
sib child bothpar	follow foster institut immig	47,600 households in 1990; 9,400 children (age 12+) in 1990	Every 6 months for 36 months
sib		15 million in 1990	Decennial (cross-sectional)

TABLE 1 Continued

Survey	Family Material Resources	Family Process	Contextual Data
National Health Interview Survey — Child Health Supplement	income welfare hlthins	marhist	move

Family Material Resources

income: summary measures of family income
source: sources of family income are identified
welfare: welfare receipt
hlthins: health insurance coverage
assets: family assets
tenure: whether rent or own home
month: income data reported on a monthly basis
year: income data reported on a yearly basis
multi: income data reported every few years

Family Process

time: amount of time spent by parent(s) with child
activty: activities between parent and child
ppcnflct: conflict between parents
pccnflct: conflict between parent(s) and child
soccap: social capital measures (e.g., extended kin and community contact(s)
rules: house rules for child regarding homework, television watching, bed time, dating, etc.
commun: frequency, styles and/or content of communication between parent and child
violnce: reports of physical violence within the family
spend: family spending patterns
marhist: parental marital histories
deprsn: parental depression measures
biopar: all biological parents of child within household are identifiable

Survey Characteristics

Special Advantages	Special Problems	Sample Size	Periodicity
black absparent exact	institut immig	17,110 children in 1988	1981, 1988 (cross-sectional)

Contextual Data

neighhd: measures of neighborhood characteristics
school: measures of school and/or classroom characteristics (e.g., curriculum, student body demographics)
zip: zip code level data available, or zip code identified
county: county-level characteristics available, or county identified
state: state-level data available, or state identified
peer: information on peers of child (e.g., characteristics, attitudes)
move: residential mobility history

Special Advantages

sibs: siblings are included in the sample and identified
Black: Black oversample
Latino: Latino oversample
Asian: Asian oversample
child: child is surveyed
bothpar: both parents are surveyed, if in same household
exact: exact relationship of child to all household members is determined
tract: tract-level data has been appended to the survey
absparent: data on the absent (noncustodial) parent is gathered
cheval: child evaluations are performed in person or through standardized tests

Special Problems

follow: child is not followed if child moves to a new household
foster: foster children not included is sample frame, or not separately identified
institut: institutionalized children not included in sample frame
unrep: sample is not nationally representative
nopar: parents are not surveyed
immig: cannot identify children of immigrants

TABLE 2 Review of Child Outcomes Covered in Federal Surveys

		Child Outcomes By Age Group				
Survey	Birth	0-5	6-11	12-17	18-24	25+
Panel Study of Income Dynamics (PSID)	Health			cog/ed demog work income	cog/ed demog work welfare income	health cog/ed demog work welfare income
National Longitudinal Survey of Youth (NLSY)				health cog/ed behav demog work welfare income	health cog/ed behav demog work welfare income	health cog/ed behav demog work welfare income
National Longitudinal Survey of Youth—Child-Mother Data (NLSY-CM)	prenat health	health cog/ed behav presch chcare	health cog/ed behav chcare	health cog/ed behav demog work income	(future)	(future)
National Educational Longitudinal Survey of 1988 (NELS88)		presch		cog/ed behav demog work	(future)	(future)

National Survey of Children (NSC)	health		health cog/ed behav chcare	health cog/ed behav demog work welfare	health cog/ed behav demog work welfare income
Survey of Income and Program Participation (SIPP)		health chcare	health chcare	health cog/ed demog work welfare income	
National Survey of Families and Households (NSFH)		health cog/ed behav presch chcare	health cog/ed behav chcare	health cog/ed behav demog work welfare income	health cog/ed behav demog work welfare income
High School and Beyond (HS&B)				health cog/ed behav demog work	health cog/ed behav demog work welfare income
Consumer Expenditure Surveys (CEX)				work income	

TABLE 2 Continued

Survey	Child Outcomes By Age Group					
	Birth	0-5	6-11	12-17	18-24	25+
National Crime Victimization Survey (NCVS)				cog/ed work		
Decennial Census, Public Use Micro-Sample (5%)		presch		cog/ed demog work welfare income	health	
National Health Interview Survey—Child Health Supplement 1988	prenat health	health behav presch chcare	health cog/ed behav chcare	health cog/ed behav demog		

prenat: mother received prenatal care
health: health measures, general or specific
cog/ed: cognitive ability and educational attainment measures, such as standardized tests, grades, and/or years completed
behav: behavioral problems measures (such as the BPI), delinquent and pro-social activities
work: employment information such as usual hours and weeks worked, employment history, and job classifications
demog: fertility and marriage data on the child
welfare: information on welfare receipt by the child
income: income generated by the child
presch: preschool measures such as participation, cost, and type and characteristics of program
chcare: child care measures such as hours per week, type and characteristics of provider, and costs

whether they add to a child's well-being immediately, time and money are expended with the intent of enhancing the future health, cognitive ability, and productive social behavior of children.

Resources with which investments in children are made take many forms and are derived from the various systems or, to use Bronfenbrenner's term, contexts in which the child develops. We classify these as family, kin, peer, school, neighborhood, community, and larger societal systems. Societal systems include government policies that provide (or deplete) resources for children in general or for particular subgroups of children.

Decisions about resource investments are made on an almost continual basis by parents and, in adolescence, by the children themselves, in the context of changing circumstances and opportunities. Communities and the national government make decisions about institutional investments less frequently, although investments are ongoing at these levels as well.

Constraints on Choices

Choices are always constrained. No parent can expend more than 24 hours in a day for work, parenting, sleep, and leisure-time activities. A poor mother faces a difficult choice if she wants to move to a better neighborhood or school district, in that her limited income must be spent for food, clothing, and other basic needs as well as housing. A mother who is physically ill or has a mental health problem may not have the energy to invest a great deal of time in providing her child with stimulating experiences or acting in a warm and responsive manner. Parents with two or more children must divide time, money, cognitive investments, and emotional resources among the children. Not only do parents with different levels of economic and psychological resources distribute them differently, but also individual parents with the same set of constraints may also make different choices (e.g., how much time to spend with a given child).

Analogous limitations constrain choices regarding the provision of extrafamilial resources. Voters and administrators make choices about how much to spend on schools, how much to invest in programs for disadvantaged schools, how to organize and staff schools, and how much to spend on extracurricular activities. All of these influence the institutional resources invested in a given child. These constraints may influence children directly (via a school's facilities and climate for learning) as well as indirectly (via the family's investment in the schooling process itself).

Types of Family Resources and Interactions Among Resources

It is useful to concentrate on four general kinds of resources: financial, time, psychological, and human capital. Economic models have looked at the financial and time resources that are made available to the children in a family (Hill and Stafford, 1980; Lazear and Michael, 1987) and consider the human capital (e.g., schooling level) of the parent as an indicator of the likely "quality" of the parent-child interaction time. Much more is known about income than about time use. Time-use diaries have been extremely useful in describing the activities on which parents spend time and how much time is spent in child-oriented activities (Timmer et al., 1985). Despite this work, very little is known about how income and time are distributed across children within individual families—that is, how much is allocated to various household members or the process by which trade-offs between income and time are made.

Human capital includes the parents' levels of formal schooling, together with special skills, training, and other characteristics that affect financial or "psychic" income. Psychological resources at the family-system level include characteristics of the parents as well as parenting behavior. Relevant characteristics include the mental and physical health of the parents, the quality of their relationship, the psychological importance to them of factors such as education and work, and beliefs about the parental role in childrearing. Parenting behavior includes a wide range of behaviors directed toward the child as well as interactions between parent and child. Some of the most important include provision of learning and stimulating experiences, communication and decision-making styles, warmth directed toward the child, disciplinary practices, monitoring and supervision, and engagement. All of these have been shown empirically to be associated with child well-being (Maccoby and Martin, 1983; Bornstein, 1995; Holmbeck et al., 1995).

Parents vary as to their ability to provide these resources (i.e., a mother with little education may not provide many learning experiences because she herself is unable to read, a parent with little money may not be able to purchase books). Parents also make decisions that make it more or less likely that such psychological resources will be available to the child. For example, the barely literate mother might be able to enter a literacy program or be part of a family resource program that could provide such services. The poor mother may not be able to buy books, but, if the neighborhood or school has a library outreach program, she would be able to bring books into the home. Such parental decisions, however, are constrained by factors such as time availability and the resources available in the neighborhood.

Parents face choices about allocating their limited resources. Residence in a single-parent household means less parental time is available to the child (Hill and Stafford, 1980; Nock and Kingston, 1988). Residence in a stepparent household also results in less time spent in parental interaction than would be expected given the presence of two parent figures (McLanahan et al., 1991; Thomson and McLanahan, et al., 1993; Hetherington, 1993). Other adults in the household may provide the child with more time with a parental figure. For example, in multigenerational households, the grandmother or grandmother figure often functions as a coparent with regard to responsibilities and time spent with the child. Coresidence in multigenerational households presumably would offer children more resources (see Furstenberg et al., 1987; Furstenberg, 1976; Kellam et al., 1982), except in cases in which the grandparents cannot help with child care or, if ill, might require care themselves (Chase-Lansdale et al., 1994).

If both parents work, or if a single parent works, time is severely constrained. However, one would expect the addition of extra income to compensate in part for the time constraint. With greater income, from example, parents are able to purchase better-quality child care services. For families at the low end of the income spectrum, however, the loss of time due to working is probably not offset by high-quality child care, in that child care choices are constrained by income if relatives are not available (Hofferth and Phillips, 1991).

Trade-offs also involve social capital and psychological resources. If mothers who work find juggling work and parenthood stressful or unsatisfying or too much of a time drain, they may put less effort into providing stimulating experiences for their children or may exhibit less warmth toward their children (Wilson et al., 1995; Weinraub and Wolf, 1983; Lerner and Galambos, in press; Zaslow et al., forthcoming). If a mother who is residing with her own mother is not working (or bringing money into the household), conflicts may arise over the roles of both generations in the care of the children, which may be translated into less warmth or less provision of learning experiences by either the mother or the grandmother (Brooks-Gunn and Chase-Landsdale, 1995; Chase-Lansdale et al., 1994).

Types of Extrafamilial Resources

Important time and money inputs also come from institutions (e.g., schools, youth centers) outside the family. In addition, social capital has recently been conceptualized as an important potential resource (Coleman, 1988). Extrafamilial social capital consists of the interpersonal connections that families establish with people outside their immediate families. Time (e.g., helping others, volunteer work) and money invested by the family in these connections build a stock of resources that the family can call on when necessary. A neighborhood rich in connectedness among families and individuals and with high expectations for its children has a level of trust and stability that could prove extremely beneficial to children.

A study by Garbarino (1991) is illustrative. He looked at various neighborhoods in terms of child abuse and neglect rates, fitting a regression line for the rates of abuse/neglect and neighborhood income. Of special interest were neighborhoods with negative residuals—that is, neighborhoods that would be expected to have higher child abuse rates than was actually the case. These neighborhoods were characterized by stability, supportiveness, and trust—in other words, they appeared to have high levels of social capital. Overall, however, we know relatively little about how connections to the community promote child well-being.

Development and Resources

Most resource models do not take into account the age of the child or adolescent. The volume and type of resources may be more highly associated with well-being at some ages than others. For example, the spacing of births is more linked to academic outcomes during the preschool years (i.e., school readiness) than during the adolescent years (Furstenberg et al., 1987). Having many preschool children is probably detrimental because young children benefit from high rates of parental interaction; time spent with parents decreases dramatically during late childhood and even more in adolescence (Feldman and Elliott, 1990). Consequently, having many children, all of whom are young, takes away parents' ability to spend time with each of them.

Moreover, resource models do not take into account individual differences in children. An illustration may be taken from the work on low-birthweight children. Very low-birthweight children (1,500 grams or less at birth) often have difficulties in regulating moods and states. Parents who have little psychological or human capital may not be as responsive to the special needs of their biologically vulnerable child. They may not avail themselves of community services to provide themselves with better parenting skills or the child with remedial intervention. Biologically vulnerable children may be more affected by familial or extrafamilial resources than children without biological problems. Similar arguments may be made with respect to children who have emotional vulnerabilities (i.e., the child who is temperamentally difficult, shy, or active) or cognitive vulnerabilities (i.e., the child with mild mental retardation or developmental difficulties).

Current resource theories also do not explicitly consider the intersection of familial and extrafamilial resources. That is, certain families may benefit more from resource-rich neighborhoods than others (Klebanov et al., 1994; Duncan et al., 1994a). Consequently, we wish to extend our resource-based framework to include age-sensitive measures, individual differences, and context. These additions provide links between resource frameworks and existing life-course and ecological (contextual) frameworks.

CRUCIAL DESIGN FEATURES OF DEVELOPMENTAL DATASETS

The breadth of the constructs included in the various theoretical perspectives that are incorporated into a resource framework requires a range of data to test these theories. In this section we identify key elements of datasets that have proved especially useful in testing and drawing policy conclusions from the theoretical framework we advocate. We begin with examples of measures of developmental outcomes, resources, and family processes identified by theory as important. We turn next to methodological issues, producing illustrations of survey design features that have proved invaluable in implementing and estimating the models. Many of the illustrations are based on results from smaller-scale studies; all have implications for the data collection improvements we outline in this paper.

High-Quality, Longitudinal Measurement of Child Outcomes

In measuring child outcomes, the goal is to identify objective indicators of competence or well-being. No matter how objective a parent is about the characteristics of his or her child, it is difficult for anyone to judge accurately the achievements of the child across a range of behaviors. Even in an instance in which parents are asked to describe simply whether a child has achieved a particular developmental milestone, variations in parental definitions can affect outcome rankings. For example, in responding to the Social and Motor Development Scale in the 1981 Child Health Supplement of the National Health Interview Survey, mothers with graduate-level educations were more critical of their young children. And teachers in a school attended by children of highly educated parents may be more critical of an average child than a teacher would be who saw the same child in the context of a community with a lower educational level. For these reasons, it is desirable to use standardized and nationally normed measures whenever possible.

Longitudinal assessment of outcomes is desirable since how changes in resources influence children's circumstances is a question for both theory and policy. Theoretically, issues center on how malleable development is, and what boundaries constrain development (Brim and Kagan, 1980; Hunt, 1961; Lerner, 1984). Of policy relevance is also whether changes in maternal circumstances, such as education, marital status, employment, and welfare receipt, have the potential for altering children's development (Wilson et al., 1995; Brooks-Gunn, in press). Programs targeting at-risk, often poor families are typically based on the assumption that altering family circumstances will benefit children as well as parents (Huston, 1992; Chase-Lansdale et al., 1994; Palmer et al., 1988). However, without outcome data on children prior to and following a change in family resources (such as maternal movement from welfare to work, maternal completion of schooling, family enrollment in a supplemental food program) or a change in community resources (such as entrance into a Head Start program or another early education program, use of a neighborhood family resource program), it is impossible to determine whether a child outcome is due to the resource change or to unmeasured differences between families who did and did not change their circumstances or receive a community resource.[2] *Thus, direct, longitudinal assessment of child outcomes, using nationally normed tests, represents an important component of any large-scale data collection effort.*

Measurement of Age-Appropriate Outcomes

It is essential to assess child outcomes in ways that are optimal for the age and developmental stage of the child. Standardized cognitive and school achievement tests take into account the rapid changes that occur throughout the childhood and adolescent years. Even then, some tests are not appropriate over the entire first two decades of life. Infant intelligence tests are constructed quite differently from childhood tests, in part because of the limited language abilities of infants and toddlers (Brooks-Gunn and Weinraub, 1983). Intelligence tests like the Weschler series have different versions for preschool children and for older children and adolescents (WPPSI and WISC).

Instruments used in national surveys to assess cognitive ability (e.g., PPVT-R; Dunn et al., 1981) focus on one aspect of language competence—receptive language or vocabulary. Although appropriate for children from age 3 through adulthood, they may be of limited use at the younger ages, especially for children who have not had any experience with situations such as naming and pointing and for children who, because of adverse family circumstances or biological conditions, are not speaking at age 3. The Bracken Basic Concept Scale assesses school readiness and is also brief and easy to administer in a home setting, even for an interviewer untrained in psychometric testing.

School-related outcomes also are sensitive to developmental age or phase. Grade failure is not a particularly good question to ask about children in kindergarten and first grade to predict failure from earlier experiences, since school situations are often quite fluid in the early grades. Similarly, current grade repetition is not relevant for high school students, since so few are held back. Instead, dropping out of high school and school absence are better measures of academic problems during high school.

Age grading is also important for behavior and emotional problems. What is considered a problem at one age may not be at another. A good example is biting: many young children go through a phase of biting others. Consequently, behavior problem scales (parents or teachers are asked to rate the frequency or severity of a list of behaviors and feelings, typically on a 3-point scale) are usually standardized by age.

Measurement of Developmental Phases and Transitions

Ideally, data collection efforts assessing child outcomes and family resources should be designed to permit estimation of models during and through key developmental phases and transitions. Scholars of child and adolescent development differ as to how to identify a phase or a transition period, as well as on whether development is so continuous that it is meaningless to talk about phases or transitions. However, school transitions in our society mean at the very least a movement to a different organizational structure as well as a change in how family, peers, teachers, and neighborhoods relate to the child. These transitions include the transition from preschool to elementary school, the transition to middle (or junior high) school, the transition to high school, and the transition out of high school (into the work force, higher education, vocational training, or unemployment). We believe that much more work needs to focus on these transitional periods. It is clear that many children fare poorly at these transition points, which in turn undermines their life trajectories (Alexander et al., 1993; Natriello, 1987; Brooks-Gunn et al., 1993a; Simmons and Blyth, 1987). Other transitions are important to an understanding of children's development. The transition to parenthood is crucial because it sets the stage for subsequent parent-child relationships, family interchanges, and potential gender-role divisions in the care of offspring and residence with the offspring (Ruble et al., 1990; Deutsch et al., 1988; Belsky, 1984; Cowan and Cowan, 1990; Shereshefsky and Yarrow, 1973).

The experiences of the mother and her unborn child also influence the health and neurological competence of the newborn, with concerns about adequacy of prenatal care, prenatal drug use, and prenatal stress and support being paramount (Robins et al., 1993; Berendes et al., 1991; Institute of Medicine, 1985). The Child-Mother Supplement of the National Longitudinal Survey of Youth is one dataset that, by starting the study prior to childbearing of the original adolescent cohort, allows an opportunity to study this transition (Chase-Lansdale et al., 1991). Transitions that typically involve young adults (and in some cases adolescents) are not studied in great detail. We would include here the transition to a household separate from parents and parental figures and the transition into the work force (which does not always occur at the end of adolescence and high school).

Thus, in terms of national data collection efforts, *questions should be tailored to at least five age groups—the four school groupings and the infancy period—and focus on transitions between these periods as well as transitions into adulthood and parenthood.*

Multiple Domains of Outcomes

The important domains of child and adolescent outcomes include the cognitive, emotional, social, health, and school-related (Brooks-Gunn, 1990). Employment, earnings, and fertility also become important in the late teen and early adult years. Outcomes in these various domains are linked in different ways to family and community resources.

An example may be taken from the Baltimore Study of Teenage Motherhood, a 20-year longitudinal study of more than 300 young women who gave birth in Baltimore in the late 1960s, their mothers, and their children (Furstenberg et al., 1987; Brooks-Gunn et al., 1993b). Different kinds of family resources predicted school failure (grade failure by age 16 and high school dropout by age 19 to 20), early sexual experience (intercourse by age 16), and behavior problems (a scale score). Number of children in the family during the preschool years was associated with school failure but not early sexuality. And the presence of a father figure in the home during the early adolescent years was important in delaying the sexual debut but was not predictive of high school difficulties.

Another reason to include multiple domains is that, in many cases, children and youth who are not faring well in one domain are also having problems in another domain. Ongoing research is examining the ways in which adolescents' problems occur together and the sequencing of the emergence of problem behavior (Dryfoos, 1990; Jessor, 1992). Subgroups of adolescents exhibit clusters of risk-taking behaviors, and certain risk-taking behaviors show a somewhat orderly progression of acquisition (cigarette use in the elementary school being predictive of alcohol and marijuana use in the middle school being predictive of the use of other drugs in high school years; Yamaguchi and Kandel, 1984). Including a narrow range of outcomes in a study would not allow for an examination of the clustering and timing of problem behaviors. *Thus surveys should consider measuring outcomes across different domains.*

High-Quality, Longitudinal Measurement of Family Resources

Most theories of child and adolescent development view as important the overall level of family economic resources. The statistical relationship between available material resources and child well-being is well established in the literature (Kalmuss and Fenelly, 1990; U.S. Department of Health and Human Services, 1992; Duncan et al., 1994b; McLoyd, 1990;

Shaw and Emery 1987; Dryfoos, 1990; Wilson, 1987; Hill and Duncan, 1987; Mare, 1980; Brooks-Gunn et al., 1993a).

Underappreciated in much of this literature, however, is that longitudinal studies find great temporal variability in family income, both within (Survey of Income and Program Participation) and across (Panel Study of Income Dynamics) years and both within and outside the United States (Duncan et al., 1993). One-quarter of U.S. families who are poor in one year are not poor the next (U.S. Bureau of the Census, 1989), and only about one-half of children who are poor in a given year are poor over longer periods (Duncan and Rodgers, 1991). What implications does this variability have for studies of child and adolescent development?

Duncan et al. (1994a) use data from the Infant Health and Development Study to relate patterns of short- and longer-term poverty over the first five years of life to IQ at age 5. After controlling for conventional demographic and socioeconomic measures (family structure, maternal education), they find powerful associations between IQs and family income levels. Of particular interest is the finding that the IQs of ever-poor children are affected by the persistence of their poverty. Net of numerous controls, children poor on all four occasions when family income was measured scored five IQ points lower than did children in families whose income histories showed only transitory poverty. This and other research suggests a crucial role for family economic resources in models of child development (see Duncan et al., 1994a).

It should be noted that detailed assessments of family income provide a great deal of additional information on the family's situation, including welfare receipt, labor market involvement, and income-generating assets (wealth).

Accordingly, we draw two conclusions. First, in addition to conventional measures of family socioeconomic status, *high-quality measurement of family income is crucial for testing resource-based theories of child and adolescent development. And second, also important is longitudinal measurement of family income, enabling researchers to distinguish between temporary and persistently low levels of family economic resources.*

Measurement of Time Inputs

Although given a prominent place in most developmental models, measures of the quantity and the quality of time spent by parents with their children are almost never available in the kinds of datasets we review. Maternal schooling level is typically used as a measure of the likely quality of the mother's time. Mother's supply of labor outside the home is usually measured and sometimes taken as a (problematic) indicator of time not available for parenting activities. Although several surveys ask questions regarding time spent in a variety of parent/child activities (e.g., television, homework, meals, special activities), there is virtually no recent, direct measurement of parental time inputs.

Careful measurement of such time inputs was achieved in a national time-use study conducted in the late 1970s and early 1980s (Juster and Stafford, 1985). Following methodological work suggesting that time diaries are the best method for obtaining unbiased measurement of time inputs, such diaries were obtained from a national sample of adults and children.

When coupled with teacher reports of academic achievement in elementary school, the coding scheme enabled Stafford (1987) to analyze the developmental consequences of parental time spent in direct learning activities, such as reading to children, as well as other parental activities at which children were present. Although it should be kept in mind that his results are based on small samples, Stafford found highly significant effects of direct activities on academic achievement.

Time diaries on children require roughly 15 minutes of interviewing time per recalled day and are thus a time-intensive method for collecting data on parental time inputs. *Periodic comprehensive measurement of patterns of parental time use are highly desirable. Some existing national surveys should consider adding shorter question sequences that would provide at least some data on parental time inputs.*

Measurement of Family Process

Family processes or functioning are important to the health and development of children, both in their own right and as mediators of material resources and child outcomes. A recent review of the literature has identified a number of important categories of measures of family processes that affect child well-being, including communication (parent-child and parent-parent), parent-child time together and activities, degree of commitment to the family, degree of social connectedness, religious/spiritual orientation, capacity to adapt to new situations, and the existence of clear family roles (Krysan et al., 1990). In addition, family conflict and styles of parental discipline are often emphasized in this literature (Zill, 1983).

The statistical relationship between available material resources and child well-being is well established in the literature. Low income has been related to less adequate prenatal care (Kalmuss and Fenelly, 1990), low birthweight and higher infant mortality (U.S. Department of Health and Human Services, 1992), slower cognitive development (Duncan et al., 1994b; McLoyd, 1990; Shaw and Emery, 1987), higher rates of adolescent risk behaviors (Dryfoos, 1990), and lower levels of educational and socioeconomic attainment as adults (Wilson, 1987; Hill and Duncan, 1987; Mare, 1980).

Relatively little is known, however, about the processes internal to the family that can account for observed relationships between resources and outcomes.[3] Our resource model indicates that family processes will to some extent mediate the relationship between available material resources and child outcomes (see, for example, Klebanov et al., 1994). However, it is often argued that observed relationships between material resources and child well-being are in fact the result of currently unmeasured or poorly measured family processes that correlate with material resources but are not determined by them (e.g., Murray, 1984). This is an important distinction, since the policy implications are vastly different depending on how one specifies these relationships. In either case, however, the proper measurement of family processes, and their inclusion in models relating material resources to child well-being are key to a deeper understanding of the links between material resources and child well-being.

Multiple Levels of Measurement

Although studies of community influences on human behavior have a long tradition (Park et al., 1967; Wirth, 1956; Shaw and McKay, 1942), only recently have researchers successfully combined individual, family, and neighborhood-level measures in national or multisite developmental datasets. Much of this work was inspired by William Wilson's (1987) theories of social isolation as inherent in neighborhoods with particularly high concentrations of poor people.

Among the notable empirical contributions to this recent literature are Crane's (1991) and Clark's (1993) respective analyses of specially linked family-tract cross-sectional files from the 1970 and 1980 census-based Public Use Micro-Sample (PUMS) files; Brooks-Gunn et al.'s (1993b) examination of neighborhood effects in the PSID and the Infant Health and Development project; and the Garner and Raudenbush (1991) study of data, analyzed with hierarchical linear models, on a sample of children in one education authority in Scotland in the mid-1980s coupled with areal data taken from the 1981 Census of Population. In the U.S. studies, neighborhood data are usually obtained from tract-level economic and demographic data from the decennial census and matched to families' addresses.

Most U.S.-based sources have found that, after controlling for family-level resources, the presence or absence of affluent neighbors is a more powerful predictor of adolescent well-being than is the presence of low-income neighbors—a finding that supports theoretical models of neighborhood effects based on beneficial neighborhood institutions (e.g., police protection, parks, schools) rather than the "epidemic" models based on peer-induced contagion effects.[4] Given the early stage of this research, these findings should be viewed as tentative but intriguing, with much more still to be learned about the influences of neighborhood resources.

National household surveys should append neighborhood-based data to their data files. This task is often surprisingly easy, especially in the first wave of most national surveys. This is because the tract/Block Numbering Area (BNA) identifier of sampled addresses is routinely gathered as part of the sampling process.[5] It is a simple and inexpensive matter to use these identifiers to merge neighborhood characteristics (e.g., poverty rate, extent of female headship, male joblessness, ethnic composition) from STF3 decennial census data files. The resulting merged family-neighborhood files offer a rich combination of interview-generated family data and census-generated neighborhood data that can be used as independent variables in various analyses of child development.

Given their geographic detail, such merged data raise confidentiality issues.[6] In the case of census Bureau data collections, the use of these matched data could be limited to census analysts as well as outsiders serving as census fellows. As for data collections outside the federal government, the matched data could be released under special contractual conditions, such as those applicable to the PSID.

Whenever possible, *appending information regarding other extrafamilial environments, most notably school characteristics, would also be valuable.* NCES samples are generally drawn from schools, and school-level data are routinely made available in analysis files. Household-based surveys must incur more expense in gathering school-based data. When such information is drawn from a survey of the teachers of the children in these samples, the questionnaires (which can be set up to use less expensive self-enumeration) can be designed to provide information on both the achievements of the individual children and key aspects of the school environment.

There is also the possibility of asking families about key elements of their neighborhoods—danger, drugs, unemployment, etc. This would enable researchers to address the methodology question of the extent to which perceptions and tract-level variables match, as well as the more substantive issue of how perceptions and objective characteristics interact. For example, resilient families may live in bad neighborhoods and perceive them as bad, but they may then respond to these conditions with intensive efforts to monitor their children. Less resilient families may live in bad neighborhoods but not perceive them as such and therefore not engage in as much monitoring.

Measurement of School Contexts

Schools are an important extrafamilial environment for child and adolescent development. Information on school functioning can be collected from self-enumerated teacher questionnaires that are sent to the child's school after permission to contact the teacher (and the teacher's name and address) is obtained from the parent. Data that can be collected include: (1) characteristics of the child, such as school grades, school engagement, parental involvement, school absences, peer relationships/social competence, attention in the classroom, and classroom-related behavior problems and (2) school characteristics, such as social climate, ethnic mix of students (in a given classroom), and teacher experience/credentials.

In several national or multisite studies, response rates to such teacher surveys range between approximately 75 and 80 percent (e.g., National Survey of Children, Moore and Peterson, 1989; Infant Health and Development Program, Brooks-Gunn et al., 1993b; Study of Elementary School Outcomes of Low Birth Weight Children, McCormick et al., 1992). The data obtained from elementary school teachers and high school teachers are often different (e.g., high school teachers have much less contact with students) and teacher-based information on 5- to 7-year-olds is less useful than data on slightly older children, since many children in that age range have not experienced school-related problems or are experiencing transient problems that resolve themselves with emotional maturity or increased cognitive skills. By age 8 and third grade, however, school problems are predictive of subsequent school failure (Brooks-Gunn et al., 1993a; Baydar et al., 1993; Snow, 1983).

Measurement of Family Relationships

Increased attention should be placed on different household arrangements as well as changes in these arrangements. When the focus is on child well-being, national studies must document the relationship of various parents and parent figures to each child.

Most research has focused on marital or parental status, rather than on changes in households or on links between marital states and individual children (Brooks-Gunn, in press; Thomson and McLanahan, 1993). Distinctions of potential importance include: (1) stepparent families in which the father is the custodial parent; (2) stepfamilies in which the custodial mother has not been married prior to her marriage to the stepfather (often seen in the case of a never-married single mother, often a teenager, who marries later); (3) never-married single males who marry and become stepparents; (4) custodial parents who marry a third or a fourth time; (5) cohabiting adults with children; (6) biological parents who have separated or divorced and then reunited; and (7) cohabiting adults each with children from a previous marriage (Brooks-Gunn, in press).

It is most common to determine family relationships by selecting a head or reference person and then asking for the relationship between each family member and this reference person. This is not sufficient for many important purposes, since it often does not allow the researcher to distinguish important relationships among members of subfamilies. If, for example, there is a three-generation family with a grandmother, her two daughters, and the daughters' children, then the relationship "granddaughter" does not provide enough information to classify children as siblings or cousins. In fact, mothers and their children cannot always be connected. As explained in the next section, *we view as crucial the collection of information about family relationships that identifies the natural and stepparents of all children living in the household.*

Most work on family relationships has been cross-sectional in nature, not focusing on the effects of changes in these family arrangements (see, as exceptions using national longitudinal datasets in the United States and Great Britain, e.g., Baydar, 1988; Cherlin et al., 1991; Kiernan, 1992). Using a framework focusing on transitions dictates that data on family resources and child outcomes be collected over a long enough time period that sufficient numbers of family structure changes will occur (Hetherington and Arasteh, 1988; Hetherington and Clingempeel, 1992).[7]

It is important to note that transitions in family structure often cannot be inferred reliably in a longitudinal study from changes in reported marital states. A woman married in two consecutive waves may have divorced and remarried between the waves, and, even if an analyst checked for changes, measurement error in husband characteristics (e.g., age) may make it difficult to infer transitions without asking about it directly. *Longitudinal studies should ask marital and fertility histories during each wave in a way that covers the entire time interval between waves.*

Coupled with this work is a concern for the relationship of the child to the noncustodial parent as well as the resources provided to the child by the noncustodial parent (Maccoby and Mnookin, 1992; Garfinkel et al., 1995; Teachman, 1991). *It would be valuable for at least some national surveys to collect information on noncustodial parents regarding economic, emotional, and time resources.* Information on the level of child support payments awarded (if any), the level received, and the stability of receipt would be welcome additions to national data collection efforts as well (Garfinkel et al., 1995). Changes in compliance of noncustodial parents and award of payments as a result of the Family Support Act of 1988 allow for natural experiments, in that one can examine payment levels and contact with children prior to and following changes in the law, as well as state-to-state variations (see McLanahan et al., 1994, who estimated predicted child support for each state to model differences in child support enforcement policy, using data from the Current Population Survey Child Support Supplement).

Measurement of Extended-Family Relationships

There is great theoretical interest in the extent and effects of intergenerational relations, especially in the flows of time and money between children and their parents. Such flows can affect the resources available to children and the need for public resources.

We have already provided examples of instances in which young children and adolescents living with their parents receive time and some (usually undetermined) share of the family's total income. Once children enter the late teenage years, they face important decisions about postsecondary schooling, careers, and living arrangements. Transfers from parents, in the form of both time and money, are of great potential importance at this stage. When children continue to live with their parents, the bulk of transfers consist of in-kind services. Children's college attendance can be greatly facilitated if tuition payments are made by parents or grandparents. Choices about home ownership, jobs obtained through personal connections, and start-up capital for independent business endeavors can all be influenced by the financial and social capital of a child's extended family.

Although some of this information (e.g., whether any help was received with tuition payments) can perhaps be recalled reliably by the grown children, parental financial resources during the time in question cannot be addressed without reliable information on these resources gathered from the parents themselves. Thus *it would be desirable for longitudinal studies of children making the transition to adulthood to continue to collect information from parents as well as children, regardless of whether the children are still living with their parents.*

There is an added methodological benefit from such information, as illustrated by Gottschalk's (1992) analysis (based on the Panel Study of Income Dynamics) of the links between parental welfare receipt and welfare receipt by daughters as they enter their adult years. He attempts to purge the parental welfare receipt measure of its sources of noncausal correlations with daughter's receipt by using patterns of mother's welfare receipt *after* the daughter has left home to adjust for the effects of unobserved heterogeneity. His argument is that the *future* welfare use of the mothers cannot have caused prior decisions leading to possible welfare receipt on the part of daughters and therefore is a valid control variable for the heterogeneity. Only by following parents after children leave home is such an approach possible.

Natural Experiments

Alone among their disciplinary colleagues in their insistence on testing theories against real-world data, labor economists in the last decade have effected a remarkable transformation in their methodology. Structural models based on tenuous identifying restrictions and ever more sophisticated econometric modeling are being replaced by reliance on "natural experiments." We endorse this development and encourage other disciplines to consider (or, in some cases, continue) work along these lines.

Drawing on a long history of work from related disciplines, Currie and Thomas (forthcoming) use sibling data from the National Longitudinal Survey of Youth to compare the cognitive development of siblings, some of whom did and some of whom did not participate in the Head Start program. Because siblings share a similar family background (including material and social resources and aspects of genetic endowment ranging from cognitive ability to temperament and physical and mental health), a comparison of their cognitive differences constitutes a kind of natural experiment, since such differences will be largely free from the confounding effects of unmeasured family background. Geronimus and Korenman (1992) and Hoffman et al. (1993) follow a similar strategy with data from the National Longitudinal Survey of Youth, the original National Longitudinal Survey cohorts, and the Panel Study of Income Dynamics in estimating sisters' differences in adult economic and demographic status as a function of whether a given sister had borne a child during her teenage years.

More subtle natural experiments have been extracted from datasets that were never designed to be relevant for developmental research. Bronars and Grogger (1992) consider the birth of the second child in twin pairs as an exogenously induced increase in family size in estimating the effects of family size on a family's economic well-being. Only data released from the decennial census provide enough observations on twins; regrettably, Grogger and Bronars were hampered by the quality of the fertility information available in census files; still, the approach represents a creative use of secondary data to test theory.

Owing to the ingenuity of the researchers and the resulting idiosyncratic nature of the experiments, it is difficult to generalize about the literature that has made use of natural experiments. Many of these studies require very large samples, which *suggests that child development studies should be added to the many important uses of data from the decennial census in discussions of future design changes.*

Common to much of the developmental research based on natural experiments is the need for clear data on family relationships, especially in the identification of sibling pairs. As noted above, this task proves especially problematic in multigeneration households in which relationships are established between household members and the head or reference person in the household. As set out in more detail below, *unambiguous data are needed showing the relationships among all possible pairs of individuals who reside in a given family. Also, clean information on birth dates has proved valuable in much of this research.*

Random-assignment experiments are even better than natural experiments in providing exogenous variation in right hand-side measures of interest. In 1988, Congress passed the Family Support Act, creating the JOBS program to assist families receiving Aid to Families with Dependent Children (AFDC) in obtaining basic education, job training, and job search services. Because many more AFDC recipients are eligible than are or can be currently served, mothers of preschoolers were assigned either to an experimental group mandated to participate in JOBS or to a control group not so mandated. The developmental effects of this program on the preschool children of AFDC recipients are being evaluated by Child Trends, Inc., as a substudy of a much larger evaluation of the JOBS program being conducted by the Manpower Demonstration Research Corporation. *It is essential that such government experiments with significant potential to affect children be evaluated in light of the possibility of providing experimental data on child development.*

Leverage for Policy Analyses Provided by State-to-State Variation in Program Benefits and Structure

Another kind of natural experiment of special interest for policy research is rooted in the fact that states often differ from one another in the benefit levels and other key features of the social policy programs they administer. Payments to three-person families from the AFDC program ranged from $119 per month in Alabama to $688 in Alaska in fiscal 1991 (Committee on Ways and Means, 1993). Many studies have attempted to use this variation to infer what would happen to work effort or family structure if the overall level of benefits from programs such as AFDC were to be changed (Moffitt, 1992). For example, Moore et al. (1994) use state-level policy variables, such as the AFDC benefit level, state abortion policy, and the adequacy of each state's family planning coverage in an event-history analysis of the determinants of adolescents' age at first intercourse. Similarly, Garfinkel et al. (1994) examine the effect of state child support on the economic status of children with absent parents.

Common to all of these studies is the addition of a state-of-residence identifier to the household and individual-level data. *Adding state identifiers as a routine matter to all national surveys would be invaluable.* In cases in which sample sizes within smaller states are judged to be too small to preserve the confidentiality of responding families, we urge that the datasets identify as many states as possible.

Oversamples of Minority Groups

Knowledge of the development of minority children and youth in the United States is woefully inadequate (Spencer and Dornbush, 1990; Earls, 1992; Spencer et al., 1985; McLoyd, 1990; Lamberty and Garcia Coll, 1994; Garcia Coll, 1990). Furthermore, studies of minority children and youth tend to focus on problem behavior, rather than on competence or normal development. This is true even though representative samples include minorities.

Generally, the national datasets reviewed in this paper include enough African-American children and youth for separate analyses. In part, this is due to the fact that African-Americans have been oversampled in many national studies (see Table 1). At the same time, current studies do not allow for a separation of black respondents who are not African Americans (such as Caribbean blacks). Most datasets do not include enough Hispanic-American children and youth, in part because oversampling has not always been done and, unless supplemented by a fresh sample, studies begun in the 1960s and 1970s are not representative of the Hispanic-American immigration patterns of the past 15 years. And only one of the surveys we review oversampled the Asian population (see Table 1).

Another issue complicates understanding of Hispanic-American children and families. Different groups of Hispanic-Americans are quite distinct. Cultural beliefs, place of origin, geographic location in the United States, and recency of immigration all differ for Cubans, mainland Puerto Ricans, Dominicans, and Mexicans, in addition to Hispanic-Americans from other Latin American countries. Groups also differ with respect to their status in the United States and in their country of origin. For example, Cuban-Americans are unable to travel back to Cuba, whereas mainland Puerto Ricans, as citizens, have no restrictions of movement. Other Hispanic-Americans have to contend with immigration restrictions. These differences alter social support systems in this country and the country of origin. In many research situations, it is unwise to treat Hispanic-Americans as a single group.

However, with the exception of the oversampling of Cuban-American and Puerto Ricans in the Hispanic sample of the Panel Study of Income Dynamics, none of the national datasets has enough Hispanic-Americans to separate out even the two largest groups: Puerto Ricans and Mexican-Americans. *To be most useful, all new national datasets should oversample Hispanic-Americans as well as African-Americans. If resources permit, dataset designers should also consider oversampling Asian-Americans as well as Hispanic subgroups such as Puerto Ricans.*

There are also arguments in favor of oversampling on risk factors such as low-income and high-poverty neighborhoods. One, based on experience with the Panel Study of Income Dynamics, which oversampled on the basis of low family income, is that such oversampling be done using relatively *exogenous* factors, such as neighborhood conditions and parental schooling levels, rather than *endogenous* conditions, such as family income. Whereas weighing adjustments handle the endogeneity problem in theory, in practice many analyses of income dynamics opt to avoid potential problems of endogeneity by excluding the low-income oversample.

Multiple Informants

There are several reasons to obtain the perspectives of more than one person about a child and his or her family. The primary reason is that many kinds of information are known better by some persons than others. For example, young adolescents are unlikely to be as well informed regarding their family's income and asset position as a parent. And the parent is unlikely to know many, if any, details about the child's use of alcohol or drugs or about his or her sexual behavior.

The perspective of a respondent may also be skewed simply because the individual lacks sufficient distance and objectivity to make a judgment. Assessments of children's behavior by teachers, for example, tend to be considerably less positive than assessments provided by parents (Moore, 1986). Using data from the 1976 wave of the National Survey of Children, Moore found that the evaluation of the classroom teacher seems to be the better predictor of later behavior. When multiple respondents address the same questions or issues, this can help researchers address and perhaps adjust for measurement errors of various sorts.

Although obtaining data from multiple informants appears to be an expensive addition to a study, it can often be done rather cheaply. For example, in face-to-face interviews, interviewers are already in the home and can provide assessments on a wide array of topics. The biggest incremental cost of obtaining additional information often consists of the careful training of the interviewers and the coding of the observational data. Similarly, data from adolescents can sometimes be obtained by giving the adolescent a self-administered questionnaire to complete while the parent is being interviewed, or to mail back. Following up on nonresponse can increase costs, as can possible additional incentive payments. However, the increment to data quality afforded by having a second respondent is so high in some instances (such as teenage substance use, delinquency, and sexual behavior) that even a substantial additional cost is warranted.

Minimizing Attrition in Longitudinal Surveys

The utility of data from all surveys is threatened by nonresponse in their initial (or, in the case of cross-sectional surveys, only) interviewing wave. Longitudinal surveys face the problem of additional nonresponse in subsequent waves. *We view as crucial that surveys budget sufficient resources to minimize possible problems owing to attrition.* Techniques for motivating interviewers and respondents have been developed to produce response rates in the initial wave in excess of 80 percent and to keep subsequent nonresponse to no more than a few percentage points. Better still are surveys that attempt reinterviews with nonrespondents from prior waves. Some 14 years after its initial interview, the National Longitudinal Survey of Youth routinely interviews more than 90 percent of its wave-1 respondents.

Some attrition is inevitable even in the best-run longitudinal surveys. An important but neglected challenge in using longitudinal data is to gauge the impact of attrition on estimates of developmental models. It has proved almost impossible to do this since the determinants of attrition overlap extensively with the righthand-side measures in the developmental models. Helpful here would be attrition-related experimental treatments on the part of the survey organizations. For example, one might offer a monetary payment to a random portion (say, one-fourth) of the sample that was well in excess of the payment offered to the rest of the sample. This information would be very helpful in discerning the impact of attrition on the behavior of interest.

CHARACTERISTICS OF EXISTING SURVEYS

We have chosen for review 12 major federally sponsored surveys containing data on children. The surveys have been grouped into three categories: long-term longitudinal, short-term longitudinal, and cross-sectional. In keeping with our emphasis on the importance of collecting data across time, all but two of the surveys reviewed are longitudinal to some degree. Specific suggestions for improving each survey are presented in the next section.

The salient characteristics of each survey are presented in Tables 1 and 2, reflecting our criteria for good survey data on children. Table 1 summarizes available data on family resources, family processes, and extrafamilial context; special advantages and disadvantages of each survey; and sample size and periodicity.[8] Child characteristics are summarized in Table 2 by age group and, within age group, by substantive category. A complete list of possible characteristics for each column is presented at the end of each table, with brief explanations as needed.

Long-Term Longitudinal Surveys

Panel Study of Income Dynamics

The Panel Survey of Income Dynamics (PSID) has been conducted on an annual basis since 1968. In 1993, the survey involved some 7,900 households. It includes an oversample of black and Hispanic families, facilitating separate analyses of these groups. Adult family members (and their children) who leave to establish a new household are followed and included in subsequent waves. The survey collects very limited data on all children in the household. Children are interviewed only after leaving to establish their own households.

The PSID contains extensive and detailed information on family material resources; transfer income data are available on a monthly basis. It contains very limited information on family process; however, valuable information is available on family spending patterns. Census data relating to place of residence are available at the tract, zip code, county, and state levels.

Only very limited information is available concerning child outcomes before age 16, including birthweight and an occasional report of health status. Schooling, labor, and income data are recorded for all children ages 16 and older. Complete birth histories are also available for all female children age 12 and over. Children who go on to form their own households are given the full battery of survey questions.

National Longitudinal Survey of Youth

The National Longitudinal Survey of Youth (NLSY) is an annual survey begun in 1979. The original sample included over 12,000 young men and women ages 14-21. A special military subsample was included, as were oversamples for blacks, Latinos, and poor whites. Among respondents to the 1979 survey attrition has been very low, about 10 percent at the 1991 interview. As of 1994, respondents range in age from 29 to 36. Current plans are to continue the survey at least for the foreseeable future. Interviews will take place every other year after 1994.

Parents are interviewed about family income data only, and only when their children are under age 18. All other information on personal and family background is obtained in interviews with the youth. The survey is designed to look at labor force participation and the transition from school to work and so is especially useful for analyses relating to the transition to adulthood.

Information on material resources of the family of origin is extensive, but only for those respondents who were living with that family at the time of the first survey. A limited set of retrospective questions regarding the condition of the family at age 14 is available for all respondents. Process measures for family of origin are practically nonexistent, though some data might be gleaned from a special time-use survey filled out by the youth in 1981 for those youth still living at home. Available contextual data include population descriptors for county and state of residence, characteristics of the high school attended, and a few questions regarding peers. Data files with appended zip code level census data have been created and may be available on a restricted basis.

Outcome data are available in many substantive areas beginning with the first year of the survey, at which time respondents ranged in age from 14 to 21. Many measures are available on a yearly basis into adulthood (ages 29-36 as of 1994). The dataset is particularly rich in schooling and labor force data. For example, labor force activity data are available on a weekly basis beginning with the calendar year previous to the first survey in 1979. Some retrospective data regarding fertility, drug use, and high school activities are available for all respondents.

National Longitudinal Survey of Youth: Child-Mother Data

Surveys of the children of female respondents of the NLSY were begun in 1986 and continue on a biennial basis. Following the NLSY sample frame, there is an oversampling of blacks and Hispanics. All children in each family are surveyed, allowing for analyses of sibling pairs.

Although the sample of women in the NLSY is nationally representative, the sample of their children is not representative at present, since they are disproportionately the children of early childbearers. As the survey continues and children of delayed childbearers become part of the sample, it will become increasingly representative.

All of the data collected in this biennial supplement are merged with the annual data collected in the NLSY main data file. Thus, there is a considerable amount of detailed income, education, and labor force information available on the parents of these children, particularly the mothers. Family-process data are limited but include a HOME environment scale and questions relating to marital conflict. Contextual data are limited to county and state characteristics.

Through a combination of mother interview and in-home child assessment, detailed and age-appropriate measures of each child's social, emotional, cognitive, and physiological development are taken. These measures include the Behavior Problems Index, the Peabody Picture Vocabulary Test-Revised, the McCarthy Scale of Children's Abilities, and the Peabody Individual Achievement Test. In 1992, questions were added concerning television-viewing habits and how older children spend their time after school. Pre- and postnatal information is also gathered for each child.

Although plans to interview teachers have been dropped, school data are being added to the Child-Mother data file. Starting in 1994, the children of the NLSY ages 15 and over will be given a full, personal interview of the kind given to their parents when the study first began. A new NLSY cohort study is to be fielded; it will probably include some of these children of NLSY mothers in the new sample.

National Educational Longitudinal Survey of 1988

The National Educational Longitudinal Survey (NELS88) is a large, nationally representative longitudinal survey of eighth graders begun in 1988, designed to focus on school and school-to-work transitions. The survey has been taken every two years from 1988 to 1994. The next wave is planned for 1998. The initial sample size was 24,599 students from 1,057 public, private, and church-affiliated schools. The sample has been enlarged in 1990 and 1992 in order to make it representative of 10th and 12th graders for those respective years. Because of a two-stage cluster sample design that included approximately 24 children per sample school, hierarchical linear modeling (a multilevel analysis technique) can be applied to these data.

The survey includes responses to detailed questionnaires from students, their parents, several teachers, and the school administrator. Student achievement scores are also included. Parent questionnaires were left out of the 1990 wave, leaving an unfortunate gap in the data on family background.

Data on family material resources are sparse, limited to total family income and assets (parental report). Family-process measures include questions about parent-child activities and time together, rules, and patterns of parent-child communication. In 1992, questions were asked of parents regarding their intended financial contributions toward their child's postsecondary education. Contextual data are a great strength of this dataset. Detailed information regarding the characteristics of the school and the specific classes attended by the student is included. Some questions are asked about peer attitudes. Finally, census data for each school catchment area are available on a restricted basis to specially licensed data users.

Child outcomes concentrate on schooling and academic achievement and also include questions on work, prosocial and delinquent behaviors, and childbearing. Information on preschool attendance is the only retrospective child data gathered.

National Survey of Children

The National Survey of Children (NSC) is a longitudinal survey begun in 1976, with a sample of 2,301 children ages 7-11. Waves 2 and 3 (completed in 1981 and 1987) followed a large subset of these children through ages 18-22. In wave 2, the survey included all children of disrupted or high-conflict families and a subsample of the rest. The sample size at wave 3 was 1,147. No further waves are planned. Black households were oversampled. Two children were interviewed in a subsample of households (554 families in 1976), allowing for the possibility of sibling studies. Parents, teachers, and children were all interviewed. The initial wave included in-person child assessments. Similar questions are often asked of both parents and their children, allowing for interesting comparisons across respondents.

Data on family material resources are limited primarily to the year in which the interviews took place, although some retrospective information was obtained in wave 3 regarding welfare receipt and maternal employment patterns. Family income is recorded in categories. The family-process measures are the most detailed and numerous of any of the surveys reviewed here. They include measures of family activities, time together, parent-child and parent-parent communication and decision-making styles, styles of parenting, rules in the home, measures of parental conflict and violence, and detailed parental marital histories. Data on the quality of relations of both parent and child with the absent parent post-separation/ divorce are also gathered. Contextual data include characteristics of the child's school, school classes, and neighborhood, as well as zip code and state-level characteristics, including state policy measures such as AFDC benefit level.

Child outcome measures include a broad array of age-appropriate measures of physical health, cognitive abilities and achievement, emotional well-being, and social development. The data have been used most frequently to examine the impact of family processes (particularly separation and divorce) on various measures of child development.

Short-Term Longitudinal Surveys

Survey of Income and Program Participation

The Survey of Income and Program Participation (SIPP) is a continuous survey in which panels are interviewed every four months for approximately two and one-half years. It is a representative survey of the U.S. civilian noninstitutionalized population. Panels have varied in size from 13,000 to 21,500 households. The 1993 panel has 20,000 households. Because of the overlapping design, cross-sectional analyses can be produced combining two panels, doubling the sample size in many years. Members age 15 and older (and their dependents) who leave the household during the period covered by the survey are followed.

The core questionnaire, repeated every four months, asks detailed questions concerning employment, income, and participation in federal social support programs. Much of the information is collected on a month-by-month basis. Questions are asked about all adults age 15 and over in the household. Special modules covering personal history and data on school enrollment and financing are administered once or twice to each panel.

In addition, there are a number of special topical modules. Some have been asked of every panel to date; others have been fielded only once or twice. Topics include child care arrangements, child support agreements, functional limitations and disability, utilization of health care services, support for nonhousehold members, and others.

Information on family processes is very limited. Marital histories are available for parents in the household. Detailed child care information is collected concerning each of the three youngest children in the household. In addition, the child support module (asked once of each panel) gathers detailed information regarding child support agreements, payments made, and time spent by children with the noncustodial parent.

Information in the core questionnaire is gathered for all children in the household who are age 15 or older. Information beyond basic demographic information (age, sex, etc.) is generally not available for children under age 15, unless collected in a topical module such as the module on child care.

Beginning in 1996, the Census Bureau plans to change the sample design and field nonoverlapping panels of 50,000 households, to be followed for a total of 52 months. In addition, a special SIPP panel, the Survey of Program Dynamics (SPD), is being designed to last for 10 years. The SPD will make special efforts to collect data on the children in SIPP households. It will be designed as an extension of the SIPP 1993 panel.

National Survey of Families and Households

The National Survey of Families and Households (NSFH) was designed to accommodate family-oriented research on a wide variety of topics and from many research perspectives. Households were originally surveyed in 1987-1988, and again five years later. There are no plans at this time to follow up with a third wave, although respondents are being tracked, making a third wave possible. The original sample included over 13,000 households, with a total of 7,926 children represented in those households. Double samples were taken for black and Hispanic households, single-parent families, cohabiting and newly married couples, and households with stepchildren. The oversampling of less common family types makes this a uniquely valuable survey for family research.

In-person interviews were conducted with a randomly chosen adult over age 18. In addition, self-administered surveys were given to the respondent and to the spouse/partner. In the follow-up survey, brief interviews were completed with those who were focal children age 5 and over in the initial survey. Both focal children who had left the household and parents who had separated or divorced since the original survey were followed and interviewed. In addition, a parent of the main respondent was also interviewed in the follow-up survey.

A limited amount of sociodemographic and behavioral information is gathered on every child in the household. In addition, there is a much more detailed set of age-appropriate questions asked concerning a randomly selected focal child. These questions cover a broad range of outcomes in the areas of health, social development, behavior problems, and cognitive achievement. No direct assessments of the child were made in either wave of the survey, however.

Focal children were ages 0-18 at the time of the first survey. Thus, while this dataset allows one to look at a child only at two time points, five years apart, it does allow one to analyze in detail the transitions between all adjacent developmental phases, including the transition to early adulthood.

Information concerning a household's material resources is very detailed, although the data refer primarily to the status of the household and its members at the time of the survey only. Income is identified by source, and in many cases according to the person who generated it. Questions are asked concerning income flows to and from extended kin and between ex-spouses.

Family-process data are one of the great strengths of this survey owing to the breadth and the depth of information gathered. Exact relationships between the adult respondent, spouse/partner, and each of the children in the household are recorded, as are detailed marital and fertility histories of all adult respondents. Questions are asked concerning time spent and activities engaged in by the focal child and each parent (including noncustodial parents), rules, parent-child communication patterns and conflict. In addition, there are many measures of the quality of the spousal relationship, including interspousal conflict, conflict resolution styles, violence, global marriage quality, and sharing of household duties. The CES-D depression scale is also administered to all primary adult respondents.

Finally, there is a host of measures of social capital regarding the relationship between adult respondents and extended kin, friends and neighbors, and community organizations such as the church, the PTA, and recreational, civic, political, and professional groups. Some county-level sociodemographic and labor force characteristics are also included in the dataset.

High School and Beyond

High School and Beyond (HS&B) is a nationally representative longitudinal survey of high school sophomores and seniors begun in 1980, with biennial follow-ups through 1986. It has a two-stage sampling design. In the first stage, public and private high schools were chosen. The following school types were oversampled: alternative, high-performance private, Hispanic, non-Catholic private, and black Catholic private. A total of 36 sophomores and 36 seniors from each school were included in the sample design (allowing for hierarchical linear modeling). A total of 30,030 sophomores and 28,240 seniors were interviewed in the first wave. A subsample of approximately one-half of the students was included in the 1982 through 1986 follow-up surveys. A 1992 follow-up of 1,300 sophomores was also conducted. Special files are available that allow one to link twins, siblings, and friends within the file.

Questionnaires were filled out by students, school administrators, and up to four of the students' teachers. Questionnaires were also filled out by parents of approximately 10 percent of the students. In addition, standardized test results are available for all students, as are complete high school transcripts for a large subsample of the sophomore cohort.

For the 90 percent of the sample whose parents did not fill out a questionnaire, data on family material resources are limited to a categorical income variable and a question on home ownership. The parent questionnaire, however, provides data on parental income, assets, and expenses, as well as parental education and employment.

Family-process measures in this survey include measures of parental aspirations and attitudes regarding secondary education for their child and financial planning for college. Such information, however, is available only for the 10 percent of the sample whose parents filled out questionnaires. In addition, all youth respondents are asked questions concerning the degree of parental supervision of homework and whether parents usually know where the youth is at any given time.

Contextual data are limited primarily to the extensive information available on the high school. Data include enrollment, demographic breakdowns of both students and faculty, course offerings, participation in federal programs, funding sources, school discipline problems, and grading systems. Local labor market indicators for the county or metropolitan area of residence are also available. Finally, a "friends" file permits one to identify and link friends within the sample, which allows for the possibility of peer measures.

Child outcomes covered in this database include information on high school and postsecondary education measures, job training and employment history, fertility and marriage, and income. Job and employment data are arranged in an event-history format. Available cognitive test measures include vocabulary, reading, mathematics, science, writing, and civic education. Data on educational aspirations, personal attitudes, and beliefs are also included.

Consumer Expenditure Surveys

Consumer Expenditure Surveys (CEX) collect detailed data on consumer expenditure patterns. The data are used to determine the need to revise the Consumer Price Index (CPI). There are two surveys, each with a sample size of 5,000. Each is a nationally representative sample of the U.S. noninstitutionalized population. In the CEX Quarterly Interview Survey, respondents are interviewed quarterly for a total of five quarters; they are asked to report major expenditures and those that occurred on a regular basis over the preceding quarter. Examples include rent or mortgage payments, utility bills, and purchases of home appliances and furnishings. The survey is continuous, with one-fifth of the sample replaced each quarter. In the Diary Survey, respondents are asked to keep two one-week diaries in which they record smaller purchases (e.g., food, cleaning supplies, clothes).

Information on material resources is detailed, covering the amount and sources of income, assets, and tenure, as well as participation in federal social welfare programs. This is by far the most detailed survey of spending patterns collected on a representative national sample of families with children; however, family-process data are limited to spending patterns. There are no contextual measures.

Data on children under age 14 are limited to age, race, Hispanic origin, sex, and exact relationship to the respondent. Employment data are gathered for all persons age 14 and older.

National Crime Victimization Survey

The National Crime Victimization Survey (NCVS) is designed to collect data on the incidence of crime as reported by the victims of crime. The survey is very large, covering approximately 100,000 people in 49,000 households. All persons ages 12 and older in the household are interviewed. Household members are interviewed every six months for three years, for a total of six interviews. The survey is continuous, with one-sixth of the sample replaced every six months. Households that move during the period of the survey are not followed. The sample is nationally representative. In addition, representative state-level data are available for the 21 most populous states.

Data on family material resources are limited to a measure of total family income. In addition, information on Medicaid and private health insurance coverage is obtained for those who visit the hospital as a result of an injury received during a crime. Family-process data are limited to the reporting of family violence that a respondent considers to be a crime (e.g., assault, rape) and is willing to report. State and region of residence are not identified in publicly available versions of the data file.

Child outcome measures are limited to detailed reports of crimes that affect them (if they are 12 or older) or to their household (regardless of their age). This is nevertheless important and unique information on child well-being.

Cross-Sectional Surveys

Decennial Census, Public Use Micro-Sample

The Public Use Micro-Sample (PUMS) is a large sample of households drawn from the 17 percent of the population that fills out the decennial census long form. The *5 Percent Sample*, as it is called, includes detailed population and housing characteristics for over 15 million persons. A *1 Percent Sample* version is also available. Data are available for the household, for each family and subfamily within the household, and for each individual.

Data on income are fairly detailed, with income reported by source and for each member of the household age 15 and older. Home ownership is also reported; assets and health insurance are not covered. There are no family process data gathered in the census. State and county group (census-defined constellations of contiguous counties) are identified, allowing for the possibility that state and county-group characteristics can be appended to the data. In 1970, a special "neighborhood file" was produced that included sociodemographic characteristics of the neighborhood of residence. Under special arrangement with the Census Bureau, a private researcher, Rebecca Clark, created a similar file using data from the 1980 census. For reasons of confidentiality, the latter file is not publicly available.

For children under the age of 15, outcome data are limited to school enrollment. For those age 15 and older, measured outcomes include school enrollment and educational attainment, employment status and characteristics, income, welfare status, marital status, and whether they have a child of their own living with them. If there is a health condition that impedes employment, that is also recorded.

National Health Interview Survey—Child Health Supplement 1988

The National Health Interview Survey—Child Health Supplement 1988 was a special supplement to the National Health Interview Survey, an annual, cross-sectional, and nationally representative survey of the U.S. civilian, noninstitutionalized population. For this supplement, additional information was gathered for one child between the ages of 0 and 17 in every sample household containing children. A knowledgeable adult member of the household, most often the mother, served as proxy respondent for each selected child. The 1988 Child Health Supplement gathered data on 17,110 children. Black families are oversampled. A similar supplement was fielded in 1981.

Family income data are limited to total family income and welfare status. In addition, health insurance coverage is also ascertained. Family process measures include child care arrangements, frequency of contact with absent parents, maternal marital history, and habits regarding seat belt use and the regularity of children's bedtimes. Contextual data are limited to a history of residential moves.

There are extensive data related to child health, including information on the child's birth, recent accidents, injuries and poisonings, particular childhood conditions, chronic conditions, emotional and behavior problems (including a 28-item Behavior Problems Index), and use of health care services. There are, in addition, many useful outcome measures that are not directly related to health, including whether the child has repeated a grade, reasons for discontinuing school, and the presence of learning disabilities or developmental delays.

The National Health Interview Survey is currently being redesigned. Current plans call for regular occasional supplements on child health. This redesigned survey is scheduled to be fielded starting around 1996.

IMPROVING EXISTING SURVEYS

We detail below changes in existing practices or new content in large national surveys that could significantly improve them. Before launching into survey-by-survey details, we begin with some generic procedural issues for surveys.

Research on the development of children using existing data is greatly facilitated if the survey data are organized on a child-by-child basis. In terms of questionnaire construction, this means that questions should be designed to obtain information on each individual child, using questions that are developmentally appropriate. As simple as this advice may seem, it is remarkable how rarely it is followed. For example, in the SIPP: (1) Federal Food Breakfast Program and Federal School Lunch Program participation information is not gathered on individual children; (2) child care information is asked only about the three youngest children; and (3) divorce/separation visitation data are gathered only on the oldest child if not all children have the same visitation schedule. This structure produces some bizarre data patterns on children when considered in a longitudinal context. For example, child care data would be collected on the oldest of three children, but not after the birth of a fourth child. The older of two children would have a longer time series that would cease if two younger siblings were born during the panel period.

Undoubtedly, decisions to limit the number of children about whom such questions are asked are based on interviewing time constraints. However, we believe that it is far better to have at least some information available on program participation, child care, visitation, and similar activities for *all* children (and included in those children's own data records) than to have details about only some of the children. If such data are collected on a grid, data collection time requirements are minimized. If time pressures preclude obtaining some data for all siblings, child age would represent a better decision rule than using the three youngest as the criterion for some questions and other factors as the criterion for other questions. Alternatively, a focal child or two focal children per family might be selected about whom detailed information will be consistently obtained.

One hopes that computer-assisted interviewing methods will reduce the perceived need for such unfortunate restrictions, but there is little reason for them, regardless of the mode of interview. *Question sequences about children should be constructed so that the questions are asked about all children for whom they are appropriate.*

Second, repeating a point made earlier, *it is important to collect information on family relationships that allows researchers to classify families according to type (step or biological, for example) and to establish the relationships among all pairs of individuals in the household.* Gathering information about each family member's relationship to a reference person does not provide the needed information. One option, chosen by SIPP in some of its panels, is to enumerate a relationship matrix. Family members are listed down the rows and across the columns of the matrix, and the interviewer then establishes the relationship (e.g., biological parent vs. stepparent; sibling, half- or stepsibling; cousin) between each pair of individuals. This option is somewhat cumbersome, especially in large families, particularly when computer-assisted personal interviewing (CAPI) is used. An alternative being developed by the Census for SIPP and the SPD, to be administered beginning in 1996, is to ask for relationship to the reference person as well as the identity (i.e., unique ID or listing line number) of each person's mother and father if that parent is also present in the household. Additional questions allow one to identify biological, step, and adoptive parent-child relationships and to identify virtually all remaining pair relationships within the household.

Third, child-centered analyses are facilitated by the release of data files in which separate records exist for each individual child or in which the data can easily be transformed into child-specific record form. In the case of a survey such as SIPP, this should be true regardless of whether the child was actually given his or her own interview. The medium increasingly preferred by analysts is CD-ROM. Retrieval software on the CDs is also desirable; the CD-ROMs prepared for the NLSY provide a model here.

Fourth, longitudinal studies based on families or households should *develop rules for following individuals that properly track the experiences of all children.* In both the PSID and SIPP, for example, the samples are defined to include individuals who were present in wave-1 households as well as births to individuals who were present in wave-1 households. Although minor children are properly part of the sample in both studies, following the rules in SIPP and, until recently, in the PSID did not provide for minor children to be followed if they moved to a household that did not contain at least one adult sample member. This procedure is clearly a mistake because it throws away the opportunity to track a relatively small but very important group of children who live in a variety of family structures during childhood. We know next to nothing about how frequent such occurrences are or about the developmental consequences of such arrangements.

We now turn to a survey-by-survey list.

Consumer Expenditure Surveys

The CEX provides a wealth of detail about household expenditures. With a few additions it could become an invaluable source of information for opening up the black box of intrafamily resources allocation.

We make a number of suggestions to improve the organization of existing information in the CEX:

1. Collect better information on family relationships. It is crucial to know how children are related to all of the adults in the household, because analysts will want to be able to link the incomes of those persons with the expenditures for the children. The existing family relationship information should be supplemented by asking for the household-listing line number of the natural father or mother of each household member. It would also be desirable to ascertain whether children share the same biological absent parent (for a more detailed discussion, see the recommendations for the decennial census listed below).

2. Identify state of residence for as many states as possible.

3. Attach census tract data to each record and offer the data on a restricted basis. Purchases of neighborhood inputs through choice of residence are among the most important ways that parents spend money on their children.

4. The Bureau of Labor Statistics should consider creating a special child subfile to facilitate research on children. Such a file would include expenditure data on children and basic family demographic and socioeconomic data; it would include identifiers allowing researchers to easily link child records with the more complete family records in the larger CEX data file.

5. Make the data available on CD-ROM with good documentation and provide a program to facilitate data extraction such as that currently available for the NLSY.

Suggestions for low-marginal-cost additions to the data include:

1. Collect greater detail on child care expenditures. The CEX currently collects great detail on many expenditure categories but has only a single question about child care expenditures. Some details on the type of child care services that were purchased would be desirable.

2. Collect additional data on expenditures explicitly made for children. At present, expenditures on clothing are about the only such data in the survey. Additional measures might include expenditures on education (e.g., private tuition, books, classes in art, sports, and other special classes), camps, computers, and expenditures on outings, for example, to the zoo, museum, and concerts.

3. For expenditures on clothing, establish the identity of the person for whom the clothing was purchased. Most expenditures families make benefit several family members at the same time. An exception is clothing, because most clothing is purchased for an individual member, even though some of it may find its way to the wardrobes of other family members. Thus, clothing expenditures constitute a promising indicator of a family's intrafamily resource allocations.

The Decennial Census

Although cross-sectional and limited to what can be collected on a self-enumerated form, data from the decennial census have been used for a surprising number of developmental studies. Interesting developmental measures include the school and fertility status of adolescents as well as the economic and demographic characteristics of the families in which children live. Most important, of course, is the fact that the PUMS file contains massive case counts. Researchers have exploited this feature by constructing samples of very rare populations, such as twins or immigrants from different countries or regions.

It would be presumptuous to believe that child development considerations should dictate substantial changes to the census form. However, we would be remiss if we failed to propose a useful change in the way that the census form collects its household relationship data:

1. The information on household-composition collected in the census derives from the identification of the householder (the household member in whose name the dwelling is owned or rented), a listing of all other household members, and the following question for each household member: "How is this person related to PERSON 1 [i.e, the householder]?" Response categories include: (a) husband/wife; (b) natural-born or adopted son/daughter; (c) stepson/stepdaughter; (d) brother/sister; (e) father/mother; (f) grandchild; (g) other relative (specify); (h) roomer, boarder, or foster child; (i) housemate, roommate; (j) unmarried partner; (k) other nonrelative. This information could be supplemented on the long form with questions establishing whether the individual's natural father or mother live in the household and, if so, who that person is. This could be done by asking for the household-listing line number of the natural father or mother of each household member. It would also be desirable to ascertain whether children share the same biological absent parent.

2. The Census Bureau should consider restoring the marital history question, which was eliminated from the 1990 census.

3. Because the census asks only about completed schooling, it is not possible to identify children who are enrolled in but have not completed preschool. Rewording the question would allow for such identification.

4. The Census Bureau should consider producing a matched file with family and neighborhood-level data from the 1990 census that is comparable to similar files produced for 1970 or 1980. A publicly available file such as that produced with the 1970 data would be clearly preferable, but it would be also considerably more expensive to produce because it involves generating new neighborhood-level data rather than using data from identifiable census tracts. A less expensive alternative would be for the Census Bureau to create a file that simply matches existing tract data to household records and make it available to researchers on a restricted basis.

5. The Census Bureau should consider creating family-level records in addition to household and person records for their PUMS microdata files, as is currently done for the Current Population Survey.

The National Crime Victimization Survey

The National Crime Victimization Survey is one of the largest ongoing surveys carried out by the federal government. Its information on crime victimization makes it a uniquely valuable resource for researching the well-being of adolescents and young adults (children below age 12 are not interviewed). There are a number of changes that would greatly enhance the value of this underutilized data set for scholarly research.

We make one suggestion to improve the organization of existing information for this survey:

1. Continue to create longitudinal files containing data on all seven interviews over the three-year period during which households participate. At present there is only one such file available for surveys having taken place in the period 1987-1990.

Suggestions for low-marginal-cost additions to the data include:

1. Expand the income and demographic data collected on all members of the household, which are currently minimal in this survey. Such improvements would include more detailed income and employment data, identification of the exact relationships among all respondents in the household, an expanded Hispanic-origin question to allow for the separate identification of major Hispanic subgroups, and welfare receipt. Data for children under the age of 12 (currently limited to age, sex, race, and national origin) should be expanded to include exact relationship to adults in the household and the grade in which they are currently enrolled.

2. Append state identifiers and tract-level census data to each record and make the resulting file available on a restricted basis. State laws and neighborhood conditions are of particular interest to those who study crime. At present, neither state nor region of residence is identified on the public file out of concern that victims may be identifiable because of the rarity of some crimes.

3. Ask follow-up questions concerning the disposition of crimes reported in previous waves; at present they are not. This would enhance the utility of the crime data substantially.

Suggestions for higher-cost additions to the data include:

1. Follow families who move out of the household. Currently, data for all seven waves of the survey are available only for those who do not change their place of residence. The Bureau of Justice Statistics has been considering doing this for some time and is monitoring the experience of the SIPP survey, which does follow families.

2. Gather data on the criminal victimization of children under age 12. The physical and sexual abuse of young children is far too common and too important to be ignored in a major survey of crime victimization. We realize that there are many problems in gathering accurate data of this sort

for children under age 12, particularly in the context of a telephone interview. Serious thought should be given to a special module on the victimization of children under age 12, to be administered in the home to a large subsample. Alternatively, it may be useful to ask retrospective questions of respondents ages 12-17 about incidences of assault or abuse at earlier ages.

National Educational Longitudinal Survey of 1988

The NELS88 survey contains many of the characteristics that we have identified as desirable for a dataset to study child and adolescent development. Parents, teachers, administrators, and the students themselves are all interviewed. Detailed information on school and neighborhood characteristics is available. The respondents are interviewed regularly over the course of their transition from adolescence to early adulthood.

A number of improvements could have been made to this survey earlier on (for example, the fielding of a parent questionnaire for the 1990 and 1994 waves, more detailed family income and process measures). At present, the main opportunity for improvement would be to discard current plans to skip the 1996 wave, which will leave a four-year gap between the third and fourth waves of the survey. This four-year spacing between interviews during what is for most youth the key transition period to adulthood (ages 20-24) substantially weakens this dataset for studying the transition to adulthood in general and the school-to-work transition in particular. Reinstating the 1996 wave would be highly desirable. We have been informed by Department of Education personnel working on this survey that, at this late date, intervention by the secretary of education would be required to reinstate the 1996 wave. Recognizing that there are substantial financial constraints involved, we would therefore propose that a telephone survey be considered for a 1996 wave.

In addition, it would be desirable for the current survey to be continued in some form until at least the year 2002, when respondents will have reached approximately 28 years of age. Many adult attainment measures, particularly earnings and work patterns, do not stabilize until that age. It is important that researchers be able to relate the rich information available in this dataset to stable and long-term adult socioeconomic outcomes.

National Longitudinal Survey of Youth (1979 Cohort)

In 1994, respondents in this survey ranged in age from 29 to 36. It is important that this cohort continue to be followed, at least for the next 5 to 10 years in order to continue to track important developments in fertility, earnings, and other important adult outcomes. Given financial constraints and problems associated with the accuracy of retrospective data, continuation of the NLSY as an annual survey would have been preferable, switching to telephone administration to save costs. However, given that the decision to move to a biennial format has already been made, we agree with current plans to continue with in-person interviews.

National Longitudinal Survey of Youth—Child-Mother Data

The child mother data supplements to the NLSY have proved very useful to policy scholars in child development, economics, sociology and demography (Brooks-Gunn et al., 1991). They could be enhanced by a number of relatively low-cost additions:

1. Augment information on parental relationships. It is difficult to determine the relationship between each child in a home and a residential father. Likewise, more information should be collected on noncustodial fathers about child support (financial, time, and psychological) as well as conflicts (also financial, time, and psychological) between the parents about the child.
2. Add more detail on the adolescent years as children of the NLSY age, paralleling what is known about the mothers during their own adolescent years.
3. Add more detailed information on mental and emotional health, collected from teachers, child, and mother (supplementing existing questions).
4. When these children reach their early twenties, data could be collected by telephone to reduce costs, with only occasional in-depth personal interviews.

There were plans to interview the teachers of children of the NLSY. It is our understanding that the Bureau of Labor Statistics discarded these plans out of concern that teachers would be able to look up sensitive information on one of their students and their parents. A number of federally collected or sponsored datasets have managed to collect sensitive parent and child data and conduct teacher interviews without experiencing confidentiality problems, including the National Educational Longitudinal Survey of 1988 and the National Survey of Children. We urge the bureau to develop ways in which teacher data could become part of NLSY data collection.

National Longitudinal Survey of Youth—A New Cohort?

It appears that the Bureau of Labor Statistics has secured funding for a new set of NLSY cohorts. Since the 1979 NLSY cohorts have proved to be such a valuable source of data for developmental studies, we offer some suggestions about the design of the new panel.

Although data collected from the adolescents ages 14-21 who constituted the 1979 panel have also been used for many developmental studies of individuals in late adolescence and early adulthood, the 14-21 range is far from optimal for such studies. A key problem is the lack of arguably "exogenous" information for the period prior to the time when outcomes are assessed. Many of the processes that affect adolescent development begin in early adolescence or before. Owing to limits on the accuracy of retrospective recall, concurrent data collected from, say, a cohort of 19-year-olds will have little of the rich parental background information available from individuals in a younger age range initially observed while they were still living with their parents. Data on attitudes and expectations of the youth are also problematic, since, if gathered for the first time from 19-year-olds, such data reflect the influence of endogenous decisions already taken by the youth.

If, for example, age 16 is considered to be the point at which major decisions regarding schooling and fertility are first taken, then the 14-21 age span provides only two cohorts—age 14 and age 15—for causal analyses. (Indeed, a number of analyses of teenage fertility have limited their samples in precisely this way.) Thus, starting with a younger age range would increase the sample size for causal modeling of school, family, and work transitions in youth and early adulthood.

From the perspective of sibling-based analyses, an initial sample that includes ages older than about 18 introduces a problematic set of possible biases. Although some 18-year-olds live in their own households, most still live with their parent(s). Data on independent 18-year-olds living on their own will not be accompanied by observations on younger siblings in the chosen age range since those younger sibling will, by and large, still be living with parents. (It would be possible to find the parental families and interview such siblings, but that would be expensive.) Also, 18-year-olds regardless of living arrangements are unlikely to have older siblings still living with them. The younger the age range, the less severe are these possible problems.

We view sibling-based problems in the NLS samples as important, since sibling observations are a great strength of the data set, and we predict that growing numbers of analysts will rely on the natural experiments inherent in sibling comparisons to control for heterogeneous family effects. Coincidentally, sibling observations are also much cheaper than observations on children in separate families, since only one set of parental data needs to be gathered and it often takes only one personal visit from an interviewer to gather the necessary information from all siblings. Our proposal for a new sample maximizes the number of sibling observations.

These considerations argue for a younger age range in the new NLS, with an upper age limit of 17-18 and beginning at age 12 or younger. The Bureau of Labor Statistics and the National Institute for Child Health and Human Development should seriously consider combining the need for a younger NLS age cohort with the need for a new national survey of children (discussed below) by combining the samples into a single, dwelling-based sampling frame. Detailed longitudinal information should be gathered on two of the children, with some information gathered on all children in the household. This would result in a large, nationally representative sample of children ages 0 through 18. The combined sample would represent a very broad age range, be clustered within families to reduce interviewing costs, provide abundant observations on siblings, and provide data from a "whole child" perspective. Such a survey should be conducted on an annual basis; to reduce costs, a personal interview could be conducted every two years, with telephone interviews in between.

National Survey of Families and Households

The NSFH offers the most comprehensive picture of the American family available in ongoing federal surveys. Information on material resources, family processes, family relationships, and nonresident kin is particularly rich.

We make a number of suggestions to improve the organization of existing data:

1. Release data from the second wave on CD-ROM as soon as the data are ready for public distribution. Current plans call for distributing the data on CD-ROM one year after the initial release of the data on 9-track tape. We believe that this unnecessarily restricts early access to this very rich data set. When errors have been reported and corrected over the course of the first year, a corrected CD can be produced and distributed at little additional cost.
2. Offer with the CD-ROM a customized data extraction program similar to that already available for the NLSY. Although there are fewer waves of data, the records for this data set are very complex, particularly for the second wave. This is a moderately costly undertaking, but it would enhance the accessibility of the data significantly.

Suggestions for low-marginal-cost additions to the data include:

1. Append tract-level data for place of residence and offer the resulting file on a restricted basis. Although there are important confidentiality issues here, a similar arrangement currently exists for data from the PSID.

The high quality of the family-level data in the NSFH makes tract-level data even more valuable.

2. If a third wave of data is collected, make arrangements to append social security earnings data to the files. This was attempted in the second wave; subsequently, however, Social Security personnel declined to allow the records search. Since such arrangements have been worked out for the Health and Retirement Survey, it would be worthwhile to reexamine this issue for the third wave.

One suggestion for a higher-cost addition to the data is as follows:

1. Collect a third wave of data in 1997-1998. This would offer three data points over a 10-year period covering a variety of developmental periods for children. The National Survey of Children, which had three waves also spaced five years apart, has been the basis for important research on child well-being from a developmental perspective. Every effort should be made to maintain the highest response rate possible for a third wave.

National Health Interview Survey—Child Health Supplement

The large sample size of the National Health Interview Survey makes it an important source of data about American children. However, the breadth of data available regarding the physical and mental health of children and their families, particularly regarding the factors that enhance or undermine the development of children, has been minimal. The augmented information about children provided by the 1981 and 1988 Child Health Supplements made the NHIS far more useful for understanding the occurrence of such conditions as behavior problems, chronic health conditions, and accidental injuries, as well as aspects of the child's environment related to health such as child care, school adjustment, and academic success. Data from the Child Health Supplements to the NHIS have been extensively used by researchers and provide the beginning points for time-series data analysis, if a new supplement is implemented in the next several years.

The National Health Interview Survey is currently undergoing a substantial redesign. Redesign plans call for an annual core survey to be supplemented by both periodic and occasional supplements on special topics. Current plans call for a special child supplement to be carried out in 1996 if additional funds can be secured, a matter that will be settled soon. If funding is not forthcoming at this time, it would be preferable to reschedule the child supplement rather than drop it.

For the design of the supplement, adding siblings to the sample would increase the sample size and provide for sibling analyses. In addition, data collection from teenagers themselves would enable information to be obtained on topics about which parents are poorly informed, such as the substance use and sexual activity of their adolescent children.

Information on family processes should also be obtained, particularly those that affect a range of health outcomes, such as the health-related behaviors of children, treatment obtained for health conditions, the preventive health care obtained for children, the risk-taking of children, and the differences in health status and behavior across children in a family. In addition, it is important to collect sociodemographic information specific to the children for whom health data are being collected, such as the exact biological relationship between the child and the parents in the home, contact with the absent parent, insurance coverage for the child including coverage provided by an absent parent, and any transfer income or child support payments made on behalf of that child.

The National Center for Health Statistics should adopt questions that will allow researchers to identify exact relationships between each child and their parent(s) within the household (i.e., natural, step, adoptive), both in the occasional child supplement and in the annual core survey. The National Center for Health Statistics has plans to test the relationship matrix used in SIPP, but it has tentatively decided to use a less rigorous set of relationship questions out of concern that the SIPP matrix is too cumbersome. The Panel Study of Income Dynamics has adopted an approach that identifies for each child the survey line number of each parent in the household and their exact relationship. From this information, exact relationships between each child and all other household members can be unambiguously constructed in most cases.

Finally, if funding were made available to conduct longitudinal data collection based on the child supplement, prospective analyses of the factors that lead to improvements or declines in health-related behavior, accidents, illness, and risk-taking could be carried out.

Panel Study of Income Dynamics

The PSID has gathered more than 25 years of data on the family and neighborhood environments of its representative sample of children and adolescents, most of whom have been observed since birth. No other data source comes close to assembling such a high-quality longitudinal time series on family and neighborhood resources. Lacking in the PSID, however, are outcome measures on children prior to age 16. Also lacking are family-process measures.

We make two suggestions to improve the organization of existing information in the PSID:

1. Extend to the current interviewing wave the "relationship file" that

the PSID has constructed for the years 1968-1985, showing year-by-year pairwise relationships and coresidential status of all pairs of individuals associated with the same original wave-1 family.

2. Develop and make available at minimal cost retrieval software that enables analysts to assemble data subsets and codebooks easily. Although the PSID data are now routinely released on CD-ROM, such software does not exist.

Suggestions for low-marginal-cost additions to the data include:

1. Addition a supplement to the regular telephone interview with parents, asking for outcome measures such as grade failure and behavior problems on the part of their children.

Our suggestion for higher-cost additions to the data is as follows:

1. Incorporate an NLSY-type personal interview to be conducted with all PSID families with children, in which the cognitive abilities of children and mothers would be tested, behavior problem reports on the children would be gathered from the mothers, and time-use activities would be reported by the mothers (in the case of younger children) or by the children themselves (in the case of older children and adolescents).

Survey of Income and Program Participation

The unique strength of SIPP lies in its rich and detailed recording of data on income and program participation. For analyses of the development of children, however, SIPP currently provides very limited information. To conduct causal analyses of child well-being, data are needed on child outcomes and on the family processes that translate resources into child outcomes. In addition, a broader array of resources needs to be measured than the set of income and program participation measures currently available.

In terms of child outcomes, at present children's health and educational attainment are the only outcomes available for study. It is proposed that measures of children's cognitive development and behavior be obtained in the Survey of Program Dynamics (the extended panel planned to follow the 1993 SIPP sample through the year 2002). With the addition of a broader array of child outcomes and family resources, combined with a longitudinal design, multivariate causal analyses can be conducted to examine how varied types of investments translate into attainment. That is, researchers and policy makers can assess the independent and interdependent effects of income by source, program participation, and family influences on children's education, employment, income, and family formation through childhood and into the early to mid-twenties. Moreover, it will be possible not only to extend the time period during which child outcomes are assessed, but also to expand the range of the independent variables that are examined. For example, beyond point-in-time or short-term estimates of welfare receipt or poverty, the implications of spending many years on welfare or in poverty can be compared with the implications of a brief spell of welfare receipt or poverty.

Examining income and program participation longitudinally represents an important expansion in research potential. Beyond this, an expansion in the range of resources measured is also needed. The only resources that are currently measured in SIPP are financial resources and human capital. Time inputs, the parents' psychological resources, and social capital resources in the community are not currently measured. In the absence of measures of these constructs, the only factors that can be examined as determinants of children's development and well-being are measures of income, program participation, and the structural characteristics of the family, such as family size and the number of parents present. The absence of a full set of resource measures can lead to erroneous conclusions about the role of these factors. For example, knowing only about income without knowing about the time parents spend interacting with their children could lead to an inflated assessment of the importance of money relative to other family inputs.

However, even with rich data on resources and child outcomes, there remains a gap in SIPP with regard to information on those family and community processes through which resources affect children's development, for example, family processes such as monitoring, communication, discipline, teaching, modeling of work, substance use, and marital behaviors. Addition of measures of these constructs would add immeasurably to SIPP in that the linkages through which poverty and program services affect children could be explored.

The addition of contextual information about the census tract of residence would also add to the utility of this data base, as is true for most national surveys.

Despite its many strengths, one disadvantage of SIPP is the relatively small sample size. Efforts to minimize attrition and to follow any children who leave the household are essential. Also, expansion of the sample size to 50,000, as currently planned, will enhance the utility of SIPP for the study of children.

Given the rich longitudinal information already being collected with SIPP on income and program participation, the incremental cost involved in adding measures of child outcomes, family processes, time inputs, and social capital is modest relative to the base cost of fielding SIPP. The incremental information will be extremely valuable for developmental research.

A NEW SURVEY OF CHILD AND ADOLESCENT DEVELOPMENT?

Taken as a whole, our list of proposed additions to the many national data collection projects we review is long and expensive. Unfortunately, available funds are probably insufficient to support all of these augmentations and also fund a new national survey of children. Accordingly, it is also important to consider whether it would be better to allocate resources in a piecemeal fashion across existing surveys or to attempt to pool those resources and spend a substantial fraction of them on a new survey focused exclusively on child and adolescent development.

Our suggestions for no-cost and low-cost additions to existing surveys are clearly our top priority. However, considering the trade-offs between the high-cost additions to existing surveys that we consider and the fielding of a new survey of child and adolescent development, in our judgment a new survey is the best use of available resources. The primary reason for this conclusion is that, although many of the existing datasets are likely to provide very valuable information on child development, these existing studies were either designed for other purposes or are designed too narrowly to serve as a general resource for research on children.

Specifically, among the overtly developmental data sets: (1) none of the NCES datasets covers the important period between birth and the beginning of school; none provides comprehensive data on siblings; and all are focused on very narrow cohort ranges; (2) the NLSY-Child-Mother supplement sample never represents a well-defined population of children in any given year and will not represent certain subgroups (e.g., adolescents born to older mothers) for more than a decade; and the NLSY Hispanic subsample is no longer representative due to heavy in-migration since 1979; (3) SIPP's proposed supplements on child development are ambitious, but the total amount of interviewing time available in the SIPP survey, focused as it is on income and program participation, will never be enough to provide comprehensive measures of outcomes and family process. Also, Census Bureau restrictions on data release make it difficult to add and analyze important contextual information, and the agency's perspective regarding the gathering of sensitive but important outcome and process measures unduly restricts survey content.

Also, most databases funded by a given federal department necessarily (and understandably) tend to emphasize the topics and processes of concern to that department. Yet what is needed is a data collection effort focused on the "whole child," that is, a survey that obtains information on multiple domains of well-being and factors that contribute to development across these domains.

Our list of important design features of a new study of child and adolescent development includes the following:

1. A new national survey of children should be longitudinal, with interviews at least every other year (and, if possible, every year), an initial personal interview, and regular subsequent personal interviews aimed at gathering high-quality developmental data.

2. It should contain a national probability sample of at least 30,000 children under age 18 and expectant parents, with oversampling among blacks and Hispanics, probably drawn from a dwelling-based sampling frame.[9] Asians should also be oversampled if resources permit, although their level of geographic dispersion makes oversampling relatively more expensive. A case count of 30,000 children amounts to roughly 1,500 cases per single year of age. The longitudinal nature of the file will produce a steady flow of new cases into a given age range each year; after five years, for example, roughly 7,500 children will have been observed making the transition into school.

Included in the sample should be institutionalized children who would otherwise reside in the sampled dwelling. All children should be followed regardless of subsequent institutional status or living arrangements. Proxy information should be gathered on all older siblings of sample children.

We have considered several options for drawing the sample for such a survey, each with its own advantages. One option for this survey is to draw a fresh sample of 30,000 children. A second option is to take all PSID children under age 18 and augment them to bring the total sample to 30,000. The PSID sample would supply approximately one-fourth of the total sample. The second option offers the advantage that longitudinal data from the PSID could be merged with the new survey data for the PSID portion of the sample, significantly enhancing its value for research. A third option, discussed earlier, is to expand the age range of a new NLS cohort to cover all children younger than (or including) age 18, with BLS funding data collection on adolescents and data collection among younger children funded by another agency or agencies.[10]

A fourth option is to build on SIPP's plan to add child development data to its 10-year Survey of Program Dynamics sample. Some 14,000 children could come from this source, with the SIPP core and supplemental questions providing many of the measures we advocate. Although the Census Bureau has shown an increasing willingness to consider questions on child development topics, its attitude regarding the gathering of the sorts of potentially sensitive information that must be part of any new survey of child and adolescent development prevents us from recommending SIPP as the preferred vehicle for such a survey at this time. This in no way reflects on the value of adding regular child modules to SIPP or the SPD, however. We heartily endorse the value of the SPD and of making child development an important focus of SIPP and the SPD.

3. At least some developmental and family-process data should be collected on *all* children, including very young ones. For time-consuming outcome measures in households with three or more children, 2 siblings should be randomly selected, with oversampling of twins. Information should be gathered about all important domains, with a sufficient number of questions within each domain to ensure reliability of measurement, but no single domain consuming a disproportionate share of interviewing time.

4. Parents should be asked for their permission to conduct periodic teacher interviews and to gather social security earnings histories.

5. The design should include interviews from multiple informants, including parents, children, and teachers. Interviewer observation data should also be included.

6. Neighborhood information from the most recent census should be matched to the family-level survey data.

7. A new set of cohorts should be initiated at least every decade. At a minimum, the new cohorts should be chosen to represent children born since the initial wave of the survey. Sibling-based studies would profit from a somewhat more complicated design, in which newly born siblings of original sample children are added at birth, and the fresh cohort selection should be designed to overrepresent newborns without siblings in the original cohort range. Alternatively, one may wish to opt for a continuous survey design, with a new cohort of newborns added each year.

8. Some consideration should be given to the possibility of adding on community-based intensive or observational studies of comparable samples of children. The national survey would provide the quantitative instruments and other procedures; local samples could supplement these data with richer process and contextual data.

9. There should be a vigorous competition for design and field work among coalitions of researchers and survey organizations, both private and public. The process by which the Health and Retirement Survey was begun could serve as a model for this process.

Ideally, resources for studying children and families would be available to fully augment existing surveys *and* for fielding a new national survey of children. If sufficient resources are not available to meet both of these goals, we would give priority to the low- and moderate-cost augmentations we have outlined and dropping some or all of the high-cost augmentations in favor of a new national survey of children as described above. The actual costs associated with each of these proposals should be estimated to facilitate future decision making on these issues.

ACKNOWLEDGMENTS

The authors shared equally in the preparation of this paper and are listed in alphabetical order. Work on the paper was supported by the workshop's sponsors and by the National Institute of Child Health and Human Development's Family and Child Well-Being Research Network, of which Brooks-Gunn, Duncan, and Moore are members. Two of the authors are affiliated with datasets reviewed in this paper: Moore with the National Survey of Children and Duncan with the Panel Study of Income Dynamics. In addition, Child Trends, Inc., and Brooks-Gunn are part of a consortium of organizations that have bid to design the Department of Education's Early Childhood Longitudinal Survey.

In writing this paper we have drawn freely upon a number of earlier efforts: Moore et al. (1994), Haveman and Wolfe (1994), Moore (1993), Watts and Hernandez (1982), Zill (1989), and Zill et al. (1984). We are indebted to Deborah Phillips for helping us conceptualize our task and to helpful comments from Don Hernandez, Gary Sandefur, Terry Adams, Dorothy Duncan, Valerie Lee, Susan Mayer, Robert Moffitt, Bruce Taylor, Diane Hansen, Dennis Carol, Susan Mayer, Jennifer Maddens, Michael Pergamit, Felicia LeClere, and the NICHD Research Network on Family and Child Well-Being.

NOTES

1. There are several exciting new federal data collection efforts, currently in the planning stages, that are not reviewed in this paper. The Department of Education intends to fund an Early Childhood Longitudinal Educational Study. This is to be a large, school-based, nationally representative, longitudinal survey of kindergarten children. A second effort, recently funded by the National Institute of Child Health and Human Development, is a National Longitudinal Study of Adolescent Health. This survey has as its goal to provide a better understanding of the complex forces that promote good health and those that increase risk among the nation's adolescents.

2. Randomized trials allow for an estimation of the effects of a particular treatment, in this case a family or community resource. However, in many cases involving federal or state programs, it is impossible to conduct randomized trials (see, for example, the paucity of such research in the literature on Head Start and the Supplemental Food Program for Women, Infants, and Children; McKey, 1985; Zigler and Muenchow, 1992; Lee et al., 1990; Rush et al., 1980). In addition, when community-level resources are the target of intervention, randomized trials are often not appropriate (i.e., randomizing communities is difficult, since the sample size is based on communities, not individuals, and communities are usually not comparable on all the possible dimensions of interest).

3. In an analysis of the determinants of cognitive test scores of 3-7-year-olds, Moore and Snyder found that mother's education and poverty status were not sig-

nificant predictors once controls for mother's score on the Armed Forces Qualification Test and measures of the home environment (as measured by the HOME scale), which were highly significant, were included.

4. Both Brooks-Gunn et al. (1993a) and Clark (1993) find that measures of affluent neighbors are more important than measures of low-income neighbors. Crane (1991) interprets his neighborhood measure (the percentage of workers in professional or managerial occupations) in terms of epidemic models, but it clearly measures the presence or absence of affluent neighbors. In one exception, Brown (1990), using the 1970 U.S. Census Neighborhood PUMS file, found evidence consistent with an "underclass neighborhood" or epidemic hypothesis for both white and black females when looking at teen nonmarital births and for white females when looking at high school completion. Evidence for white and black males regarding high school completion and idleness was not consistent with such hypotheses, however.

5. It is considerably more expensive to geocode addresses beyond wave 1 in longitudinal studies, since address matching would be involved and it is impossible to match addresses to census geocodes without at least some tedious map work. There would be substantial value in this additional geocoding. But the greatest value, especially given its low cost, would be in geocoding the wave 1 addresses and matching STF3 census data to these addresses.

6. One valuable piece of neighborhood information that could be distributed more widely is a scrambled version of the tract/BNA identifier. Clustered samples typically select several families per block (or adjacent blocks). It is analytically very useful to be able to sort children into groups—(1) same family (i.e., siblings), same neighborhood; (2) different family, same neighborhood; and (3) different family, different neighborhood—even if the actual characteristics of the neighborhoods are not known. These groups form the basis of an analysis-of-variance type of accounting of family and neighborhood effects. To perform this kind of analysis, one need not know any of the actual characteristics of the neighborhoods, but only whether survey families share the same neighborhood. Although this analysis-of-variance accounting capability would be quite useful analytically, it is less valuable than and no substitute for the actual decennial census measures matched to the family- and individual-level survey data.

7. An example of the importance of studying different family structures as well as the processes within families is the well-documented fact that the movement from a traditional family structure to a single-parent structure (divorce) results in less optimal functioning across domains. However, the effect is not just due to a single-parent household, in that remarriage, and the entrance of a stepparent, do not alter substantially the well-being of children (Hetherington, 1993; McLanahan et al., 1991; Garfinkel and McLanahan, 1986; Kiernan, 1992).

8. For more detailed descriptions of each survey, consult Child Trends (1993).

9. Possible national sampling frames include census-based dwellings and list-based schools. The former provides national samples of noninstitutionalized families and children; the latter national samples of school-age children. The former clusters children within neighborhoods and families; the latter within schools. As already noted, clustering provides analytic advantages in the form of sibling, neighbor, and classmate comparisons. Choice of sampling frame depends on the value of covering preschool children (which is part of dwelling but not school-based frames)

as well as the comparative advantages of clustering by siblings and neighbors versus classmates. Although we see some arguments for school-based clustering, there is greater analytic value in clustering by family and neighbor and in coverage of preschool children.

10. A new cohort of the NLSY will be fielded in spring 1996. All adolescents ages 12-17 in the household will be interviewed and followed over time; however, there are no plans to interview children age 11 or younger.

REFERENCES

Alexander, K.L., D.R. Entwisle, and S.L. Dauber
1993 First-grade classroom behavior: Its short- and long-term consequences for school performance. *Child Development* 64(3):801-814.

Baydar, N.
1988 Effects of parental separation and re-entry into union on the emotional well-being of children. *Journal of Marriage and the Family* 50:967-981.

Baydar, N., and J. Brooks-Gunn
1991 Effects of maternal employment and child-care arrangements in infancy on preschoolers' cognitive and behavioral outcomes: evidence from the children of the NLSY. *Developmental Psychology* 27(6):932-945.

Baydar, N., J. Brooks-Gunn, and F.F. Furstenberg, Jr.
1993 Early warning signs of functional illiteracy: predictors in childhood and adolescence. *Child Development* 64(3):815, 829.

Belsky, J.
1984 The determinants of parenting: a process model. *Child Development* 55(1): 83-96.

Berendes, H., S. Kessell, and S. Yaffe, eds.
1991 *Advances in Low Birthweight: An Interactional Symposium.* Washington, D.C.: National Center for Education in Maternal and Child Health.

Bornstein, M., ed.
1995 *Handbook of Parenting.* Hillsdale, N.J.: Erlbaum.

Brim, O.G., and J. Kagan
1980 *Constancy and Change in Human Development.* Cambridge, Mass.: Harvard University Press.

Bronars, S., and J. Grogger
1992 The Economic Consequences of Teenage Childbearing: Results from a Natural Experiment. Paper presented at the National Institute for Child Health and Development Conference on outcomes of early childbearing, Bethesda, Md., May 1992.

Bronfenbrenner, U.
1979 Contexts of child rearing: problems and prospects. *American Psychologist* 34:844-850.

Brooks-Gunn, J.
in press Research on step-parenting families: integrating discipline approaches and informing policy. In A. Booth and J. Dunn, eds., *Step-Parent Families with Children: Who Benefits and Who Does Not?* Hillsdale, NJ: Erlbaum.
1990 Identifying the vulnerable young child. Pp. 104-124 in D.E. Rogers and E. Ginzberg, eds., *Improving the Life Chances of Children at Risk.* Boulder, Colo.: Westview Press.

Brooks-Gunn, J., and P.L. Chase-Lansdale
1995 Adolescent parenthood. Pg. 10 in M. Bornstein, ed., *Handbook of Parenting.* Hillsdale, N.J.: Erlbaum.

Brooks-Gunn, J., G.J. Duncan, P.K. Klebanov, and N. Sealand
1993a Do neighborhoods influence child and adolescent behavior? *American Journal of Sociology* 99(2):353-395.

Brooks-Gunn, J., G. Guo, and F.F. Furstenberg, Jr.
1993b Who drops out of and who continues beyond high school?: a 20-year study of black youth. *Journal of Research in Adolescence* 3(37):271-294.

Brooks-Gunn, J., P.K. Klebanov, F.R. Liaw, and D. Spiker
1993c Enhancing the development of low-birth-weight, premature infants: change in cognition and behavior over the first three years. *Child Development* 64(3): 736-753.

Brooks-Gunn, J., E. Phelps, and G.H. Elder
1991 Studying lives through time: secondary data analyses in developmental psychology. *Developmental Psychology* 27(6):899-910.

Brooks-Gunn, J., and M. Weinraub
1983 Origins of infant intelligence testing. Pp. 25-66 in M. Lewis, ed., *Origins of Intelligence*, 2nd Edition. New York: Plenum Press.

Brown, B.
1990 The Effect of Neighborhood Characteristics on Teen Outcomes Related to Socio-economic Attainment: In Search of the Underclass Neighborhood. Dissertation. University of Wisconsin, Madison.

Chase-Lansdale, P.L., J. Brooks-Gunn, and E.S. Zamsky
1994 Young African-American multigenerational families in poverty: quality of mothering and grandmothering. *Child Development* 65(2):373-393.

Chase-Lansdale, P. L., F.L. Mott, J. Brooks-Gunn, and D.A. Phillips
1991 Children of the NLSY: a unique research opportunity. *Developmental Psychology* 27(6):918-931.

Cherlin, A.J.
1991 On analyzing other people's data. *Developmental Psychology* 27(6):946-948.

Cherlin, A.J., F.F. Furstenberg, Jr., P.L. Chase-Lansdale, K.E. Kiernan, P.K. Robins, and D.R. Morrison
1991 Longitudinal studies of effects of divorce on children in Great Britain and the United States. *Science* 252:1386-1389.

Child Trends
1993 *Researching the Family: A Guide to Survey and Statistical Data on U.S. Families.* Washington, D.C.: Child Trends, Inc.

Clark, R.
1993 Neighborhood Effects on Dropping Out of School among Teenage Boys. Mimeo. Urban Institute, Washington, D.C.

Coleman, J.
1988 Social capital in the creation of human capital. *American Journal of Sociology* 94:95-120.

Committee on Ways and Means
1993 *1993 Green Book: Background Material and Data on Programs within the Jurisdiction of the Committee on Ways and Means.* Washington, D.C.: U.S. Government Printing Office.

Cowan, P.A., and C.P. Cowan
1990 Becoming a family: research and intervention. Pp. 1-51 in I. Sigel and A. Brody, eds., *Family Research.* Hillsdale, N.J.: Erlbaum.

Crane, J.
1991 The epidemic theory of ghettos and neighborhood effects on dropping out and teenage childbearing. *American Journal of Sociology* 96(5):1126-1159.

Currie, J., and D. Thomas

forthcoming Does Head Start make a difference? *American Economic Review*.

Desai, S., P.L. Chase-Lansdale, and R.T. Michael

1989 Mother or market? Effects of maternal employment on cognitive development of 4-year-old children. *Demography* 26(4):545-561.

Deutsch, F.M., D.N. Ruble, A. Fleming, J. Brooks-Gunn, and C. Stangor

1988 Information-seeking and self-definition during the transition to motherhood. *Journal of Personality and Social Psychology* 55(3):420-431.

Dornbusch, S.M., L.P. Ritter, and L. Steinberg

1991 Community influences on the relation of family statuses to adolescent school performance: differences between African Americans and non-Hispanic whites. *American Journal of Education* 38(4):543-567.

Dryfoos, J.G.

1990 *Adolescents at Risk: Prevalence and Prevention*. New York: Oxford University Press.

Duncan, G.J.

1992 The economic environment of childhood. In Aletha Huston, ed., *Children in Poverty*. New York: Cambridge University Press.

1991 Made in heaven: secondary data analysis and interdisciplinary collaborators. *Developmental Psychology* 27(6):949-951.

Duncan, G.J., J. Brooks-Gunn, and L. Aber

1994a *Neighborhood Poverty: Context and Consequences for Development*. New York: Russell Sage Foundation.

Duncan, G.J., J. Brooks-Gunn, P.K. Klebanov, and P. Kato

1994b Economic deprivation and early-childhood development. *Child Development* 65(2):296-318.

Duncan, G.J., B. Gustafsson, R. Hauser, G. Schmauss, H. Messinger, R. Muffels, B. Nolan, and J. Ray

1993 Poverty dynamics in eight countries. *Journal of Population Economics* 6(3): 215-234.

Duncan, G., and D. Hill

1989 Assessing the quality of household panel survey data: the case of the PSID. *Journal of Business and Economic Statistics* 7(4):441-451.

Duncan, G.J., and W. Rodgers

1991 Has children's poverty become more persistent? *American Sociological Review* 56:538-550.

Dunn, L.M., et al.

1981 *Peabody Picture Vocabulary Test-Revised*. Circle Pines, Minn.: American Guidance Services.

Earls, F.

1992 Not fear, nor quarantine, but science: preparation for a decade of research to advance knowledge about the control of violence in youth. Pp. 104-121 in D.E. Rogers and E. Ginsberg, eds., *Adolescents at Risk: Medical and Social Perspectives*. Boulder, Colo.: Westview Press.

Eccles, J.S.

1983 Expectancies, values and academic behaviors. In T.J. Spence, ed., *Achievement and Achievement Motives: Psychological and Sociological Approaches*. San Francisco: Freeman.

Elliot, D.S., S. Huizing, and D.S. Agetin

1985 *Explaining Delinquency and Drug Use*. Beverly Hills, Calif.: Sage Publications.

Feldman, S.S., and G. Elliott, eds.
1990 *At the Threshold: The Developing Adolescent.* Cambridge, Mass.: Harvard University Press.

Furstenberg, F.F., Jr.
1976 *Unplanned Parenthood: The Social Consequences of Teenage Childbearing.* New York: The Free Press.

Furstenberg, F.F., Jr., J. Brooks-Gunn, and S.P. Morgan
1987 Adolescent mothers and their children in later life. *Family Planning Perspectives* 19:142-151.

Garbarino, J.
1991 Not all bad developmental outcomes are the result of child abuse. *Developmental Psychopathology* 3:45-50.

Garcia Coll, C.T.
1990 Developmental outcome of minority infants: a process-oriented look into our beginnings. *Child Development* 61(2):270-289.

Garfinkel, I., and S. McLanahan
1986 *Single Mothers and their Children: A New American Dilemma.* Washington, D.C.: Urban Institute Press.

Garfinkel, I., S. McLanahan, and P. Robins, eds.
1994 *Child Support Reform and Child Well Being.* Washington, D.C.: Urban Institute Press.

Garner, C.L., and S.W. Raudenbush
1991 Neighborhood effects on educational attainment: a multilevel analysis. *Sociology of Education* 64:251-262.

Geronimus, A.T., and S. Korenman
1992 The socioeconomic consequences of teen childbearing reconsidered. *Quarterly Journal of Economics* 107:1187-1214.

Gottschalk, P.
1992 The intergenerational transmission of welfare participation, facts and possible causes. *Journal of Policy Analysis and Management* 11(2):254-272.

Haveman, R., and B. Wolfe
1994 *Succeeding Generations: On the Effects of Investments in Children.* New York: Russell Sage Foundation.

Hernandez, D.J.
1993 *America's Children: Resources from Family, Government, and the Economy.* New York: Russell Sage Foundation.

Hetherington, E.M.
1993 An overview of the Virginia Longitudinal Study of Divorce and Remarriage: A focus on early adolescence. *Journal of Family Psychology* 7:39-56.

Hetherington, E.M., and J.D. Arasteh, eds.
1988 *Impact of Divorce, Single Parenting, and Step-Parenting on Children.* Hillsdale, N.J.: Erlbaum.

Hetherington, E.M., and W.G. Clingempeel
1992 Coping with marital transitions: a family systems perspective. *Monographs of the Society for Research in Child Development* 57(227):2-3.

Hill, C.R., and F.P. Stafford
1985 Parental care of children: time diary estimates of quantity, predictability and variety. Pp. 415-437 in F.T. Juster and F.P. Stafford, eds., *Time, Goods, and Well-Being.* Ann Arbor, Mich.: Institute for Social Research, Survey Research Center.

1980 Parental care of children: time diary estimates of quantity, predictability and variety. *Journal of Human Resources* 15:219-239.

Hill, M.
1992 *The Panel Study of Income Dynamics: A User's Guide.* Beverly Hills, Calif.: Sage Publications.

Hill, M., and G.J. Duncan
1987 Parental family income and the socioeconomic attainment of children. *Social Science Research* 16:39-73.

Hofferth, S.L., and D.A. Phillips
1991 Child care policy research. *Journal of Social Issues* 47:1-13.

Hoffman, S.D., E.M. Foster, and F.F. Furstenberg, Jr.
1993 Re-evaluating the cost of teenage childbearing. *Demography* 30:1-14.

Holmbeck, G.N., R.L. Paikoff, and J. Brooks-Gunn
1995 Parenting of adolescents. In M. Bornstein, ed., *Handbook of Parenting.* Hillsdale, N.J.: Erlbaum.

Hunt, J.M.
1961 *Environment and Experience.* New York: Roland Press.

Huston, A., ed.
1992 *Children in Poverty.* New York: Cambridge University Press.

Infant Health and Development Program
1990 Enhancing the outcomes of low-birth-weight, premature infants. *Journal of American Medical Association* 263:3035-3042.

Institute of Medicine
1985 *Preventing Low Birthweight.* Washington, D.C.: National Academy Press.

Jessor, R.
1992 Risk behavior in adolescents: a psychosocial framework for understanding and action. In D.E. Rogers, and E. Ginsberg, eds., *Adolescents at Risk: Medical and Social Perspectives.* Boulder, Colo.: Westview Press.

Juster, F. Thomas, and F.P. Stafford, eds.
1985 *Time, Goods and Well-being.* Ann Arbor, Mich.: Institute for Social Research, Survey Research Center.

Kalmuss, D., and K. Fennelly
1990 Barriers to prenatal care among low-income women in New York City. *Family Planning Perspectives* 22(5):215-218, 231.

Kellam, S.G., C.H. Brown, and M.E. Ensminger
1982 The long-term evolution of the family structure of teenage and older mothers. *Journal of Marriage and the Family* 44:539-554.

Kiernan, K.
1992 The impact of family disruption in childhood on transitions made in young adult life. *Population Studies* 46:218-234.

Klebanov, P.K., J. Brooks-Gunn, G.J. Duncan
1994 Does neighborhood and family affect mother's parenting, mental health, and social support. *Journal of Marriage and the Family* 56(2):441-455.

Krysan, M., K.A. Moore, and N. Zill
1990 Research on Successful Families. A report on a conference sponsored by the Assistant Secretary for Planning and Evaluation, U.S. Department of Health and Human Services.

Lamberty, G., and C. Garcia Coll, eds.
1994 *The Reproductive Health of Puerto Rican Women Residing on the U.S. Mainland and the Growth and Development of Their Children.* New York: Plenum Press.

Lazear, E.P., and R.T. Michael
1987 *Allocation of Income within the Household.* Chicago: University of Chicago Press.

Lee, V., J. Brooks-Gunn, E. Schnur, and T. Liaw
1990 Are Head Start effects sustained? A longitudinal comparison of disadvantaged children attending Head Start, no preschool, and other preschool programs. *Child Development* 61:495-507.

Lerner, J.V., and N.L. Galambos, eds.
in press *The Employment of Mothers during the Childrearing Years.* New York: Garland Press.

Lerner, R.M., ed.
1984 *On the Nature of Human Plasticity.* New York: Cambridge University Press.

Liaw, F., and Brooks-Gunn, J.
1994 Cumulative familial risks and low-birthweight children's cognitive and behavioral development. *Journal of Clinical Child Psychology* 23(4):360-372.

Maccoby, E.E., and J.A. Martin
1983 Socialization in the context of the family: parent-child interaction. Pp. 1-102 in P.H. Mussen and E.M. Hetherington, eds., *Handbook of Child Psychology: Socialization, Personality, and Social Development.* New York: John Wiley and Sons.

Maccoby, E.E., and R.H. Mnookin
1992 *Dividing the Child: Social and Legal Dilemmas of Custody.* Cambridge, Mass.: Harvard University Press.

Mare, R.D.
1980 Social background and school continuation decisions. *Journal of the American Statistical Association* 75(370):295-305.

McCormick, M.C., J. Brooks-Gunn, K. Workman-Daniels, J. Turner, J., and G. Peckham
1992 The health and development status of very low birth weight children at school age. *Journal of American Medical Association* 267:2204-2208.

McKey, R.H., L. Condelli, H. Granson, B. Barrett, C. McConkey, and M. Plantz
1985 *The Impact of Head Start on Children, Families, and Communities.* Final Report of Head Start Evaluation, Synthesis and Utilization.

McLanahan, S., N.M. Astone, and N.F. Marks
1991 The role of mother-only families in reducing poverty. Pp. 51-78 in A.C. Huston, ed., *Children in Poverty: Child Development and Public Policy.* Cambridge, Mass.: Cambridge University Press.

McLanahan, S., J.A. Seltzer, T.L. Hanson, and E. Thomson
1994 Child support enforcement and child well-being: greater security or greater conflict? In I. Garfinkel, S. McLanahan, and P. Robins, eds., *Child Support Reform and Child Well-Being.* Washington, D.C.: Urban Institute Press.

McLoyd, V.C.
1990 The impact of economic hardship on black families and children: psychological distress, parenting, and socioemotional development. *Child Development.* 61:311-346.

Moffitt, R.
1992 Incentive effects of the U.S. welfare system, a review. *Journal of Economic Literature* 30(1):1-61.

Moore, K.A.
1993 Children and Families: Data Needs in the Next Decade. Invited presentation given at the Interagency Family Data Workshop Group Meeting. Washington, D.C., May 25.

1986 Children of Teen Parents: Heterogeneity of Outcomes. Final Report to the Center for Population Research, National Institute of Child Health and Human Development, Department of Health and Human Services, grant # HD18427-02. May.

Moore, K.A. and Peterson, J.L.
1989 Wave Three of the National Survey of Children: Description of Data. The Consequence of Teenage Pregnancy. Final report prepared under NICHD and ASPE/ DHHS Grant #HD21537.

Moore, K.A., and N. Snyder
1991 Cognitive attainment among firstborn children of adolescent mothers. *American Sociological Review* 56:612-624.

Moore, K.A., D.R. Morrison, and D.A. Glei
1994 Welfare and adolescent sex: the effects of family history, benefit levels and community context. *Journal of Family and Economic Issues.*

Murray, C.
1984 *Losing Ground.* New York: Basic Books.

National Commission on Children
1991 *Beyond Rhetoric: A New American Agenda for Children and Families.* Washington, D.C.: National Commission on Children.

Natriello, G., ed.
1987 *School Dropouts: Patterns and Policies.* New York: Teachers College Press.

Nock, S.C., and A.W. Kingston
1988 Time with children: The impact of couples' work-time commitments. *Social Forces* 67:59-85.

Palmer, J., T.M. Smeeding, and B.B. Torrey, eds.
1988 *The Vulnerable.* Washington, D.C.: Urban Institute Press.

Park, R.E., E.W. Burgess, and R.D. McKenzie
1967 *The City.* Chicago: University of Chicago Press.

Robins, L.N., J.L. Mills, J. Brooks-Gunn, and C. McCarthy
1993 Effects of in utero exposure to street drugs. *American Journal of Public Health* 83:1-32.

Rosenbaum, J.E., and S.J. Popkin
1991 Employment and earnings of low-income blacks who move to middle-class suburbs. Pp. 342-356 in C. Jencks and P.E. Peterson, eds., *The Urban Underclass.* Washington, D.C.: The Brookings Institution.

Ruble, D.N., J. Brooks-Gunn, A.S. Fleming, G. Fitzmaurice, C. Stangor, and F. Deutsch
1990 Transition to motherhood and the self: measurement, stability, and change. *Journal of Personality and Social Psychology* 450-463,

Rush, D., Z. Stein, and M. Susser
1980 A randomized controlled trial of prenatal nutritional supplementation in New York City. *Pediatrics* 65:683-697.

Rutter, M.
1985 Family and school influences on cognitive development. *Journal of Child Psychology and Psychiatry* 26(5):683-704.

Shaw, C., and H. McKay
1942 *Juvenile Delinquency and Urban Areas.* Chicago: University of Chicago Press.

Shaw, D.S., and R.E. Emery
1987 Parental conflict and other correlates of the adjustment of school-age children whose parents have separated. *Journal of Abnormal Child Psychology* 15(2):269-281.

Shereshefsky, P., and L. Yarrow
1973 *Psychological Aspects of a First Pregnancy and Early Postnatal Adaptation.* New York: Raven Press.

Sigel, I.E., ed.
1985 *Parental Belief Systems.* Hillsdale, N.J.: Erlbaum.

Simmons, R.G., and D.A. Blyth
1987 *Moving into Adolescence: The Impact of Pubertal Change and School Context.* New York: Aldine de Gruyter.

Smeeding, T.M., and B.B. Torrey
1988 Poor children in rich countries. *Science* 242:873-877.

Snow, C.E.
1983 Literacy and language: relationships during the preschool years. *Harvard Educational Review* 53(2):165-189.

Spencer, M.B., G.K. Brookins, and W.R. Allen
1985 *Beginnings: The Social and Affective Development of Black Children.* Hillsdale, N.J.: Erlbaum.

Spencer, M.B., and S. Dornbusch
1990 American minority adolescents. In S. Feldman and G. Elliot, eds., *At the Threshold: The Developing Adolescent.* Cambridge, Mass.: Harvard University Press.

Stafford, F.P.
1987 Women's work, sibling competition, and children's school performance. *American Economic Review* 77:972-980.

Stinnett, N., and Defrain
1985 *Secrets of Strong Families.* Boston: Little, Brown, and Co.

Swithart, J.
1988 Characteristics of Strong Families. Unpublished paper, International Family Center, Logos Research Institute.

Teachman, J.D.
1991 Who pays? receipt of child support in the United States. *Journal of Marriage and the Family* 53(3):759-772.

Thomson, E., and S. McLanahan
1993 Family structure and child well-being: Economic resource versus parental behavior. Presented at the Annual meeting of the American Sociological Association. Washington, D.C., August.

Timmer, S., J. Eccles, and K. O'Brien
1985 How children use time. In F. Thomas Juster, and F. Stafford, eds., *Time, Goods and Well-being.* Ann Arbor, Mich.: Institute for Social Research.

U.S. Bureau of the Census
1989 Transitions in income and poverty status: 1984-1985. *Current Population Reports*, Series P-70, No. 15-RD-1. Washington, D.C.: U.S. Department of Commerce.

U.S. Department of Health and Human Services
1992 *Child Health USA '92.* DHHS Publication No. HRSA-MCH-92-6. Washington, D.C.: U.S. Government Printing Office.

Watts, H.W., and D. Hernandez
1982 *Child and Family Indicators: A Report with Recommendations.* Report of the Advisory Group for Child and Family Indicators of the Advisory and Planning Committee on Social Indicators. Washington, D.C.: Social Science Research Council.

Weinraub, M., and B.M. Wolf
1983 Effects of stress and social supports on mother-child interactions in single- and two-parent families. *Child Development* 54:1297-1311.

Werner, E.E., and R.S. Smith
1982 *Vulnerable But Not Invincible: A Longitudinal Study of Resilient Children and Youth.* New York: McGraw Hill.

Wilson, J.B., D.T. Ellwood, and J. Brooks-Gunn
1995 Welfare to work through the eyes of children: the impact on parenting of movement from AFDC to employment. In P.L. Chase-Lansdale and J. Brooks-Gunn, eds., *Escape from Poverty: What Makes a Difference for Children?* New York: Cambridge University Press.

Wilson, W.J.
1987 *The Truly Disadvantaged: The Inner City, the Underclass, and Public Policy.* Chicago: University of Chicago Press.

Wirth, L.
1956 *The Ghetto.* Chicago: University of Chicago Press.

Yamaguchi, K., and D.B. Kandel
1984 Patterns of drug use from adolescence to young adulthood: II. Sequences of progression. *American Journal of Public Health* 74(7):668-672.

Zaslow, M.J., K.A. Moore, N. Zill, and M.J. Coiro
in press *Implications of the JOBS Program for Children.* Washington, D.C.: Urban Institute Press.

Zigler, E., and S. Muenchow
1992 *Head Start: The Inside Story of America's Most Successful Educational Experiment.* New York: Basic Books.

Zill, N.
1983 Divorce, marital conflict, and children's mental health: research findings and policy recommendations. U.S. Senate, Committee on Labor and Human Resources. *Broken Families: Hearings Before the Subcommittee on Family and Human Services*, Washington, D.C.: U.S. Government Printing Office..

Zill, N., ed.
1989 Research and Policy Uses of Federal Data on Children and Families. Recommendations from the Second Interagency Conference on Child and Family Statistics, Washington, D.C., March.

Zill, N., J.L. Peterson, and K.A. Moore
1984 Improving national statistics on children, youth, and families. A report on recommendations made at the Interagency Conference on Child and Family Statistics, September.

Children's Transition to School

Sandra L. Hofferth

The importance of caring for and preparing children well during their preschool years so that they can learn and grow emotionally into happy, healthy, and productive adults has been well documented (Copple et al., 1993). Although particular policy concerns seem to come and go like the latest movie, there are several that are not new and appear to be lasting. Aggressive, violent, and antisocial behaviors by children shock us almost daily and crime and violence constitute the number one public issue. The increasing proportion of unmarried teenagers bearing children while still in high school is an anomaly in our highly technological society and sets us apart from the European nations. The proportion of children who do not develop the skills to be able to function adequately in this increasingly complex world continues to concern us. We suspect, although we do not know, that antisocial and precocious behavior among children living in poor families, including delinquency, violent behavior, early sexual activity and out-of-wedlock childbearing, and school problems do not suddenly emerge full-grown at adolescence. Rather, many of the diverse problems manifested in adolescence are suspected to have common antecedents in childhood behavior problems and may have common origins. In addition, skills developed in childhood can make the difference between productive, self-sufficient adults and adults who remain dependent. Because skills are cu-

Sandra L. Hofferth is at the Institute for Social Research, University of Michigan.

mulative, failure to develop these skills early makes it hard to keep up with one's classmates in school.

Children's readiness for school has been conceptualized as "the capacity to engage actively in the learning process" (Copple et al., 1993) and as "an emerging facility to experience and shape one's environment" (National Task Force on School Readiness, 1991). Whether children arrive on their first day and every day thereafter at their fullest potential depends on factors that predate their birth, including prenatal care and maternal health habits, access to health care and exposure to high-quality care and preschool programs during their preschool years, a warm and stable family, a safe and supportive community, as well as an engaging and responsive school environment (Copple et al., 1993). Thus the transition from preschool to school encompasses the period from gestation through the primary grades. This paper takes as its focus, therefore, children from birth (or during gestation) to about age 12 or 13, the end of the elementary school years.

The paper first outlines the basic scientific issues that need to be addressed by those concerned with school readiness and the transition to school. Second, it lists the federal statistical data sources that are currently available and how they address these basic issues. Third, it reviews efforts in the planning stages. Fourth, it addresses gaps in federal data collection efforts, taking into account efforts either under way or planned. A set of approaches to addressing the gaps follows. Finally, the potential role of the National Research Council in integrating and coordinating federal statistical efforts is discussed.

BASIC SCIENTIFIC ISSUES/THE BIG QUESTIONS

How Well Are Children Doing?

Documenting how well or poorly children are doing is valuable, because it raises public awareness about these problems and leads to support for interventions. Probably the most commonly addressed question is: How well are children doing?

Developmental outcomes are often categorized into three groups: (1) cognitive, (2) socioemotional, and (3) physical health (see for example, Entwisle, 1992; Powell, 1992). Goals 2000 has added (4) approaches toward learning and (5) language usage to the set of categories (National Education Goals Panel, 1993).

Cognitive

Cognitive domains include physical knowledge about objects, relational knowledge, and social conventional knowledge (National Education Goals Panel, 1993). Under this rubric I also include verbal and written language and approaches to learning. Some of the more common measures of cognitive domains include the Peabody Picture Vocabulary Test, a test of receptive language, scores on math and reading achievement tests, and scores on tests measuring memory and attention. Learning predispositions may differ by gender, temperament, and cultural patterns and values. Learning styles include curiosity, task persistence, reflection, and imagination. Tests measuring temperament are available (Baker et al., 1993). Although I am not aware of tests, I have seen teacher ratings used to measure learning styles. Finally, as an alternative measure of cognitive outcomes, behavioral measures of progress and success in school, such as retention in grade, special education placement, grades, and school dropout, are used.

Socioemotional

Socioemotional dimensions of development can be divided into emotional development and social development (see National Education Goals Panel, 1993). Self-concept is a key aspect of social and emotional development. "Self-concept consists of the traits, habits, abilities, motives, social roles, goals, and values that define how we perceive ourselves (National Education Goals Panel, 1993:14)." The ability to express feelings constructively is an important aspect of emotional development. Social interactions with adults and peers are crucial aspects of social development. One widely used measured of socioemotional development, the Child Behavior Problems Index, captures both social adjustment and emotional problems and has been widely used. Many of these behaviors are negative; positive aspects of children's behavior need to be defined and measured as well. Researchers have recently become interested in the development of moral judgments in children. However, such concepts are not yet well defined.

Health

Health includes physical development and physical abilities (National Education Goals Panel, 1993). Young children's height and weight can be measured against national norms on growth charts. Measures of birthweight, gestational age, and birth length relative to the norm are also important indicators of health (Korenman et al., 1994). Physical abilities include gross motor skills, fine motor skills, oral motor skills, and functional performance. Tests have been developed to measure the development of children from birth through school entry. This should become an even more important area. In order to obtain federal funds, special needs children are required to be identified and served at earlier and earlier ages. However, since motor development proceeds at varying and uneven rates, it may be difficult to determine the long-term implications of relatively small delays in mastering these skills.

Good health is generally identified by the lack of poor health: the lack of activity limitations, accidents, untreated chronic conditions. More work is needed to define physical fitness and good health. For example, good health habits and knowledge about risky behaviors such as smoking, drinking, and unprotected sexual intercourse are important.

Assessment Age

An important question is the earliest age at which one can first assess children's development. The Peabody Picture Vocabulary Test, for example, a measure of receptive language, is not designed to assess children before age 3. Although there are tests to measure language skills earlier, there is evidence that early cognitive assessments may not be as reliable, valid, or stable as later ones (Baker et al., 1993). Health and nutritional status may be better measured before age 3. For example, recent work (Korenman et al., 1994) finds that measures of early child health are related to cognitive assessment scores and to behavior problems. Consequently, researchers often limit assessments prior to age 3 to physical health, motor skills, and nutritional status.

What Are the Inputs Children Receive?

In order to be able to succeed, children need access to resources and services—good preschools and child care providers, good schools and teachers, developmentally appropriate curricula, families with adequate incomes, good health care, and so on. Thus the next question is: What are the inputs/resources children receive?

One concern is whether children have access to safe, nutritious, and healthy environments. What are maternal habits and life style before and after birth? Does the child receive the proper immunizations and well-child visits prior to school (Zill and Schoenborn, 1990)? A second concern is about the decline in exclusive care by parents and increased use of substitute care for even very young children (see Howes, 1992). As mothers are increasingly employed outside the home, is substitute care adequate in quality for children's optimal development? A third concern is about the decline in care by both mothers and fathers during the crucial early years of a child's life due to increasing out-of-wedlock childbearing and high levels of divorce and separation (see, for example, McLanahan, 1985, 1988; Bumpass, 1984; Hofferth, 1985). Do children receive adequate attention from both parents? A fourth concern is the increased proportion of children raised by very young, abusive, immature, unprepared, or poverty-stricken mothers with poor prospects (see, for example, Moore and Snyder, 1991; Wolock, 1981; Zill et al., 1995). Do such mothers raise children who will repeat the cycle of early childbearing, poverty, and dependence? A fifth concern is growing up in poor neighborhoods with dismal and dangerous schools (see, for example, Nettles, 1992; Karweit, 1992). To what extent do neighborhoods affect the ability of children to develop into competent, self-sufficient adults?

One line of research is to examine factors that increase the risk of failure. These, often called *risk factors*, are associated with lower success, but the mechanisms are not described. Research, again, is only suggestive, but outcomes may be linked to the economic and social conditions in which families live and the level and instability of resources available to them. These include family characteristics such as low income, minority race/ethnicity, being raised by a single mother or no parent, low birthweight, having a teenage parent, low level of maternal education, English not spoken at home, large family size, later birth order, low maternal ability, and low child ability (Hofferth et al., 1994). They also include neighborhood characteristics, such as the proportion of families in the neighborhood who are poor or female-headed and the proportion who are middle class (Duncan et al., in press).

How Do Early Experiences Affect Later Well-Being?

In order to be able to recommend solutions, we need to address the key scientific issue: How do these inputs relate to later success or failure in achieving normal physical, cognitive, and psychosocial development? Basic scientific researchers are concerned with two processes: (a) the mechanisms or paths (mediating factors) whereby children become successful or fail and programs work or do not work (Entwisle, 1992) and (b) the moderating or contextual factors, such as race/ethnicity, family and kin factors, and neighborhood (Nettles, 1992), that interact with the characteristics of children to produce varied outcomes.

Mediators

Mediating factors explain the relationship between low income, for example, and child outcomes. They include family parenting style, communication, attitudes, and beliefs (Beavers and Hampson, 1992; Powell, 1992); early childhood program participation and program characteristics (Howes,

1992); adequate nutrition, health care, and immunizations (Shonkoff, 1992); and school engagement, including appropriate attendance, completion of homework, and interest in school (Karweit, 1992).

Moderators

Moderating factors affect the relationship between inputs and outputs; they are also known as interacting factors and define subgroups for separate analyses. For example, the relationship or process may differ between boys and girls, blacks and whites, and older and younger children (Mott and Menaghan, 1993). The process may vary depending on individual parent characteristics such as warmth, on family characteristics and resources, on child temperament, on family and kin support, and on neighborhood and school characteristics.

Some subgroups in which there is special interest are children cared for by foster parents or other nonparent relatives, children with disabilities, and children of non-English-speaking parents. The latter are especially important given the debate over Chapter I funding for schools with disadvantaged students (Fix and Zimmerman, 1993) and the new requirement for schools to serve children with special needs. Do these funds make a difference? What are the appropriate ways to serve such children? Another important group consists of children not living with a natural or adoptive parent—those either in foster care or in the care of other family members. Again, this is an important group for policies such as Family Preservation and Support. Is it better to keep families together or remove them from dysfunctional homes?

Intervention/Prevention Research

Once we think we know what resources children should be receiving (in that they have been linked to later well-being), we can design intervention programs. There are three important questions:

1. *What interventions should be tried?* This type of question is directly linked to the scientific questions raised earlier. Research shows a relationship between early behavior problems and later school problems and antisocial activity. The conclusion is that early aggressive behavior is associated with later school problems; therefore, develop programs to reduce aggressive behavior (Kellam, 1993). Another example is that early childhood programs develop children's cognitive and social skills, improve health, and help parents; therefore, develop more early childhood education programs (Schweinhart et al., 1993).

2. *How effective are they?* This type of question is rarely addressed.

The Perry Preschool Project is one of the few to measure effectiveness in dollar terms (Schweinhart et al., 1993; Select Committee on Children, Youth, and Families, 1985). This permits a comparison of the returns from other types of investments. Thus the final question:

3. *What is the relative cost-effectiveness of different policy approaches/ interventions?*

For example, what is the relative payoff of:

a. Increasing direct monetary investments in children, such as immunizations and Head Start,

b. Increasing direct time investments in children, through tutoring and mentoring,

c. Increasing indirect monetary investment in children through schools and services,

d. Increasing direct monetary investment in families, such as the Earned Income Tax Credit, Aid to Families with Dependent Children (AFDC), and the Job Opportunities and Basic Skills (JOBS) programs,

e. Changing parent behavior, such as education, social services, family planning, and

f. Changing teacher behavior, through promoting developmentally appropriate activities?

The only way to address these issues is through scientific analyses that compare the relative effects of these different factors in one model. Consequently, it is important to have models that are as comprehensive as possible, that is, that include all the potential mediators.

FEDERAL STATISTICAL DATA SOURCES

Although the need for information on children has been increasing, data systems that collect needed information on children have been deteriorating. The National Maternal and Infant Health Survey program of National Center for Health Statistics will not be continued, and funds for a new Child and Family Health Supplement to the Health Interview Survey are in danger. Table 1 shows the major scientific databases on children and the scientific questions to which the data are addressed: outputs, inputs, the link between the two, and program evaluation.

Basic Scientific Issues

How Well Are Children Doing?

The major efforts at large-scale assessments of children's cognitive abilities occur under the auspices of the National Assessment of Educational Progress (NAEP). Budgeted at $29.3 million per year, NAEP undertakes major testing efforts to determine the competency levels of U.S. youth in reading, writing, math, science, U.S. history, and world geography. Whereas some information on time spent studying, reading, and watching television is collected, family demographic data are limited to those reported by students, and no information on school functioning has been obtained.

Heretofore there has been no major effort to develop a major assessment of children's socioemotional development. The National Institute of Mental Health, however, has conducted pilot studies in four sites to examine the prevalence of disorders in children from age 4 to 17 (Methodological Epidemiological Study for Children and Adolescents or MECA). This effort is planned to lead to a major set of studies in several sites around the country of the prevalence of psychiatric disorders among children and the availability and use of services in the community.

Assessment of child health has been conducted by the National Center for Health Statistics. As part of the National Health Interview Survey (NHIS), health data are collected routinely on children in the family. In 1993-1994, the National Health Interview Survey conducted a major Disability Survey, including children as well as adults (Simpson et al., 1992). In 1981 and 1988 a complete child health supplement was collected. The 1988 supplement included data on some 17,000 children from birth to age 17. Several reports have been produced using these data, and they have served as a major source of information on child health in the United States (e.g., Zill and Schoenborn, 1990). A new child health supplement has been tentatively planned for 1996; however, its funding situation is precarious.

What Inputs Are Children Receiving?

Because of government monitoring of programs, surveys for purposes of identifying who is receiving specific services are common. Of these services, early childhood programs are probably the most adequately surveyed. Studies that have obtained information on enrollments of children and about their preschool and early childhood settings include the National Child Care Survey 1990 (Hofferth et al., 1991), the 1991 National Household Educational Survey (Brick et al., 1992), the Profile of Child Care Settings (Kisker et al., 1991), the National Transition Study (Love et al., 1992), the Observational Study of Early Childhood Programs (Layzer et al.,

TABLE 1 Databases Relevant to the Transition to School

Database	Outputs			Inputs	Link Outputs/ Inputs	Inter- vention/ Evaluation
	Health	Cognitive	Socio- Emotional			
National Assessment of Educational Progress (NAEP)	X	X		X		
Methodological and Epidemiological Study for Children and Adolescents			X			
Child Health Supplements (81,88) to the Health Interview Survey (CHS)	X	X	X	X		
National Maternal & Infant Health Survey (NMIHS)	X	X	X	X		
National Household Education Survey (NHES)	X	X	X	X		
National Child Care Survey 1990 (NCCS)				X		
A Profile of Child Care Settings 1990 (PCS)				X		
Observational Study of Early Childhood Programs - Vol. 1	X	X	X	X	X	
Observational Study of Early Childhood Programs - Vol. 2				X		
National Study of Before & After School Programs (NSBASP)				X		

Survey of Income & Program Participants (SIPP)				X		
Child Care Supplement				X		
Child Well-being Module	X	X	X	X		
NCHS Immunization Surveys				X		
WIC				X		
Child Care Food Programs (CCFP)				X		
Michigan Time Use Study 1975-76 & 1982 (MTSU)		X		X	X	
Consumer Expenditure Survey (CES)				X		
NICHD Early Child Care Study	X	X	X	X	X	
National Longitudinal Survey of Youth (NLSY) Mother Child Supplement	X	X	X	X	X	
Panel Study of Income Dynamics (PSID)		X		X	X	
National Survey of Families & Households (NSFH)	X	X	X	X	X	
JOBS Child Outcomes Study (JOBS)	X	X	X	X	X	X
Prospects	X	X	X	X	X	X
Head Start - Public School Transition Study	X	X	X	X	X	X
National Transition Study				X		

1993), the National Study of Before and After School Programs (Seppanen et al., 1993), and the Survey of Income and Program Participation child care supplement (O'Connell and Bachu, 1992). The National Household Education Survey is planning an early childhood education component in its 1995 data collection wave. I do not know of a survey comparable to the Profile of Child Care Settings or the National Study of Before and After School Programs that would obtain detail on what happens in schools (although the "Prospects" study of the Department of Education has a small observational component). A prototype would be the Schools and Staffing Survey, but with observations in classrooms. The National Center for Health Statistics has been conducting state-by-state immunization surveys to monitor level of immunizations and regular surveys to monitor health promotion and disease prevention efforts for national health goals. The National Maternal and Infant Health Survey also asked questions about services (Zill and Daly, 1993). Studies have been conducted on coverage of the Supplemental Food Program for Women, Infants, Children (WIC), for example (Kotelchuck et al., 1984), and on the Child Care Food Program (Glantz et al., 1988).

Another important set of inputs comes from parents. What are children receiving in terms of care and attention from parents? What amount of time and how it is spent are questions that can adequately be addressed only through a time-budget interview that obtains a complete accounting of time spent during the day. Stylized time accounting, which asks separate questions about time spent in specific activities, is not as accurate. The 1975 and 1976 Michigan Time Use Studies are landmarks in obtaining detailed information on family members' time use. In 1981-1982, family members were once again interviewed and a time budget diary for children ages 3 to 17 was obtained (the information for children ages 3 to 5 came from parents) (Juster and Stafford, 1985; Timmer et al., 1985). The activity categories in these diaries are comprehensive. A teacher was contacted and assessments of the child's cognitive development were obtained in 1982 (Stafford, 1987). There is no comparable study currently being planned, as far as I know. The National Household Education Survey is planning a parent component in the 1996 wave. It is unlikely to use a diary approach due to its multiple objectives and limited time per household.

Several studies have attempted to define the amount of financial contribution parents make to their children—the "cost" of children. Data generally come from the Consumer Expenditure Surveys (e.g., Espenshade, 1984).

Finally, the Census Bureau is planning on adding a child well-being topical module to wave 6 of the 1993 panel of the Survey of Income and Program Participation (to be fielded in winter 1994). This primarily obtains information on parental inputs to children (child care, time spent). However, for older children it proposes to ask parents about grade repetition and school suspensions, teacher conferences due to a problem the child was having, and whether the child ever stayed out later than permitted. Health information will be obtained for all children.

What Is the Link Between Inputs and Outputs?

Although detailed data collection efforts have been made to monitor child well-being and to obtain information on inputs to children, the number of efforts that permit linking inputs with outputs is limited. Although all agencies benefit, only the National Institutes of Health, the National Science Foundation, and the National Center for Education Statistics (in the Department of Education) have these basic scientific questions as their mandate. Both the National Institutes of Health and the National Science Foundation depend on investigator-initiated projects and have severely constrained budgets. The Department of Education is limited primarily to contractual work; consequently, its flexibility is constrained, since contract work requires that the government define the scope of work as specifically as possible prior to requesting bids. Although this makes sense for some things, it does not meet the needs of scientific inquiry.

There are currently only two national surveys that follow children from preschool-age into the school years: the mother-child supplement to the National Longitudinal Surveys of Youth (NLSY-MC) and the Panel Study of Income Dynamics (PSID).

The National Institute of Child Health and Human Development (NICHD) funds the mother-child supplement to the NLSY, a Department of Labor survey. The mother-child supplement is a biennial survey, beginning in 1986, of the children of a nationally representative sample of women ages 14 to 21 when they were first interviewed in 1979. The children are assessed beginning at age 3 and interviewed directly beginning about age 10. Additional information about them is obtained from their mothers and from self-administered questionnaires. The limitations of the study are due primarily to the basic design of the Department of Labor survey rather than to the design of the child supplement. First, children become part of the survey as they are born. Thus, the older children are children of early childbearers and the younger children are children of later childbearers. As of 1990, it was estimated that the children represent about three-fourths of the childbearing of this age group of mothers. As the children age, the NLSY will eventually include children of older and younger childbearers at each age. Unfortunately, they will represent considerably different time periods and therefore may or may not be comparable. In addition, since the children are reached through their mothers, there is almost no information on the fathers of the children; however, there is more information on contact with absent fathers than with those in the household.

The richness of the NLSY lies in its assessments, along with an extensive set of background variables. The NLSY contains a basic set of assessments of cognitive, socioemotional, and physical health measures, which it has kept over the years for comparability with previous waves. Since 1986, researchers have broadened the measurement of social and emotional aspects of child functioning, but these advances are not represented in the NLSY. In addition, little information on schools and school progress is obtained.

The major drawback is that mediating factors are limited. A modified version of the Home Observation of the Environment (HOME) scale was obtained for each wave. The mental health of the mother was assessed at irregular intervals, which makes it impossible to relate to the child's well-being. In addition, almost no attitudinal information was obtained from the mother. Questions about drug and alcohol use and criminal behavior of the mother were asked only on a few occasions (although they were asked again in 1994). Assessments of the marital relationship were obtained in 1988 and 1992 only. More regular assessments would be quite helpful in linking inputs with child outcomes. As of the 1992 wave, four waves of information are available on the children, and 13 years of information are available on their mothers. Thus this survey provides a rich source of information on relatively short-term outcomes for children of income, marital status, and other family behaviors.

The Panel Study of Income Dynamics is rich at the points the NLSY is poor, in that it has detailed information throughout on both parents in households. In 1968 about 5,000 U.S. households were first interviewed. All members of these households and all the children, grandchildren, and great-grandchildren from these original sample members continue to be followed annually up to the present. More than 25 years later, about half the original sample is still being followed. Because of split-offs, in 1988 about 7,000 families were being interviewed. Since there is no mechanism for incorporating immigrants and thereby to reflect the changing composition of the U.S. population, a nationally representative Latino sample was first interviewed in 1990 and interviewed annually thereafter.

Though children are not the focus of the PSID, information on the number and ages of children in each household is obtained annually. The PSID has rich information on inputs such as family income, wealth, and labor force participation during the time the child is in the family. Moderating factors are also rich. Information on parents, family resources, and neighborhoods is available through supplements, such as on kin exchanges in 1980 and 1988, and links to the decennial censuses. Child characteristics are not available before age 16, nor were family process measures obtained. However, at age 16 and after, school enrollment and completion information becomes available. Long-term outputs after the child becomes an adult are also available, since sample children who leave home become respondents and report on their own households and well-being. The richness of the data lies in its intergenerational linkages. That is, detailed information on the families of each child is available for 25 years. Thus the data are ideal for the analysis of long-term consequences of family income and living arrangements for children.

The National Survey of Families and Households was a nationally representative sample of 13,000 households conducted in 1987. Detailed information about one focal child in each household was obtained. The first follow-up was begun in 1992. Focal children ages 5 to 18 in 1987 were interviewed by telephone in 1992-1993, when they were 10 to 23. Very little retrospective information was obtained about experiences prior to age 5. Thus this study will not be useful to follow the transition from preschool into the school-age years. However, given the richness of information collected on all household members, it may be worthwhile to create a child-based file to follow focal children over the five years of the survey to date.

Several studies have collected data longitudinally, but only during the first several years of a child's life. For example, the National Maternal and Infant Health Survey represents a national sample of women who had a live birth, fetal death, or infant death in 1988. The 1991 follow-up interviewed the families about their children 3 years after the first interview. Substantial family demographic information was obtained in this survey, including variables of interest to researchers who wish to link inputs and outcomes over the first three years.

The NICHD Study of Early Child Care originally intended to follow children for the first 2.5 years (NICHD Early Child Care Network); it now intends to follow them into first grade. This will be an enormous benefit to researchers; however, since this study is located in various sites across the country, it will not be nationally representative.

Evaluation/Intervention Studies

A considerable number of intervention programs have been evaluated. The best-known example is the Perry Preschool Project (Schweinhart et al., 1993). The data from most studies, generally small and select populations, are rarely made publicly available for secondary analysis. However, three new studies promise to provide information on the transition to school and may become available to researchers: (1) Prospects, (2) the JOBS child outcomes study, and (3) the evaluation of Transition to School programs by the Administration for Children and Families.

A major assessment of the cognitive skills and abilities of children, particularly those from low-income families, is being conducted by the Department of Education (Puma et al., 1993). This study, called *Prospects: The Congressionally Mandated Study of Educational Growth and Opportu-*

nity, will collect detailed assessments and other information for 5 years on some 30,000 students across the United States in grades 1, 3, and 7 for the purpose of evaluating the long-term effects of exposure to Chapter I services. Consequently, students in low-income schools have a higher probability of being included. Immigrant and non-English-speaking students are included in this study. An achievement test "SABE" is available in Spanish for those who prefer it, and questionnaires are also available in Spanish. Though tests and questionnaires in non-Hispanic languages are not available, the study is collecting transcripts and other information on all students. Unfortunately, because grade 1 is the first contact, very little information will be available on the transition to school. Although I do not know the actual cost of Prospects, about $9 million is budgeted for the evaluation of Chapter I programs in fiscal 1995 (Office of the President, 1994).

The JOBS child outcomes study, being conducted at three sites of the JOBS evaluation, interviewed children ages 3 to 5 at baseline, when their mothers, at intake into the program, were randomly assigned to one of three intervention groups: (1) basic educational activities, (2) employment activities, and (3) a control group. Information on the mothers and their children was obtained at baseline and will be collected 2 years after baseline when the children are ages 5 to 7. In both waves, information on the parent-child relationship, maternal well-being and characteristics, child care arrangements, and family and home characteristics, is being obtained, as well as measures of school readiness and achievement. An observational study is being conducted at one of these sites as well.

The Administration for Children and Families has a set of demonstration projects providing Head-Start-like services to assist in the transition of former Head Start children to school. Sharon and Craig Ramey, Civitan International Research Center, Birmingham, received the contract to evaluate these transition projects, the Head Start/Public School Transition Study; there are 32 demonstration projects in 31 states and the Navajo nation (Ramey and Ramey, 1993). The national evaluation project has conducted interviews with parents, teachers, and principals, along with assessments of children and classroom observations in the fall of the kindergarten year of 2 cohorts of former Head Start and non-Head Start children in randomly assigned demonstration schools and comparison schools (fall 1992 and fall 1993). All children in demonstration schools are eligible to receive services. All former Head Start children, non-Head Start children in demonstration schools, and a subsample of non-Head Start children in comparison schools in the first cohort are being followed up through at least the end of first grade in spring 1994. The original plan was to follow these children through the end of third grade; however, funding has not been provided for the third grade follow-up. Reauthorization is currently being considered.

The cost of the 32 demonstrations plus the evaluation is approximately $25-26 million per year, with about $24 million for the demonstrations and the remainder for the evaluation.

EFFORTS IN THE PLANNING STAGES

There are four studies that will potentially fill some of the gaps identified above: (1) the Program on Human Development and Criminal Behavior of the National Institute of Justice and the McArthur Foundation, (2) the Multisite Study of Mental Health Services of the National Institute of Mental Health, (3) the Early Childhood Longitudinal Survey of the Department of Education, and (4) the Survey of Program Dynamics of the U.S. Bureau of the Census.

The Program on Human Development and Criminal Behavior plans to follow 8 age cohorts of children and youth for 8 years each (Earls, 1993). The youngest cohort will consist of 1,000 females and 1,000 males beginning at age 2 or 3 and will be followed for 8 years, to age 10 or 11. A second cohort of 500 males and 500 females will begin at age 3, and again be followed for 8 years. Thus these two cohorts will provide a good picture of transition to school. The study will be conducted in 77 areas of Chicago. The outcome variables are antisocial behavior, criminality, and substance abuse. The types of explanatory variables are quite comprehensive and include most of those mentioned above.

Applications for a cooperative agreement for a Multisite Study of Mental Health Service Use, Need, Outcomes, and Costs in Child and Adolescent Populations have been requested. It is expected that the study will be conducted in several sites, including a national site, with potential follow-ups for several years. Its purpose is, first, to assess the mental health of children, as do studies of adults. Its second objective is to obtain information on the services such children receive. The National Institute of Mental Health (NIMH) conducted methodological studies of diagnostic assessments of children 4-17 (MECA); however, the assessment of children under age 4 is untested, as far as I can tell. When these assessments have received widespread validation, they should become quite useful for other surveys. The question is how they are to be validated. What are the outcomes of interest? Do these tests predict substantial problems later on? This is especially important if very young children are to be assessed, since there is apparently considerable instability of these tests measured at an early age. This series of studies links well to the Individuals with Disabilities Education Act, which requires services be provided to young children before entry into school. However, it is important to assess the relationship between scores on diagnostic tests at an early age with outcomes. Some of these measures may have a relationship to later problems; others may not.

The usefulness of these diagnostic tests is clearly important in something as potentially costly as this new legislation appears to be (Woodward and Weiser, 1994).

The Department of Education has awarded a planning contract for an Early Childhood Longitudinal Study (ECLS), with the full-scale survey planned for 1998 at the earliest. This study would follow a kindergarten cohort of children as they move into regular school to assess factors associated with normal development; it would focus on all the outcome areas described above. Substantial retrospective information prior to kindergarten would be obtained, but assessments would begin only in kindergarten.[1]

The Census Bureau has proposed a new survey: the Survey of Program Dynamics. Its objectives are to provide data showing dynamic changes in participation in welfare, health, education, and employment and training programs for 1993-2002 and in children's well-being, and to provide information to analyze causes and consequences of program participation. The sample would be drawn from the 1993 panel of the Survey of Income and Program Participation, and, when combined with SIPP data collected beginning in 1996 and ending in 2002, would provide a 10-year panel.

GAPS IN DATA COLLECTION EFFORTS

Only one national study currently in the field collects data concurrently from parents and their children both before and after entry into school and has the potential of addressing the scientific questions listed above—the NLSY-MC. This dataset has been very heavily used for this reason.

A number of gaps can be identified in the data collection efforts currently under way or planned: First, there is currently no *longitudinal study of a nationally representative sample of children starting prior to school entry*. Each of the studies that is planned or under way has either a limited age range or a sampling design that limits its generalizability. The Department of Education Early Childhood Longitudinal Study (ECLS) starts with children already enrolled in kindergarten. The National Institute of Justice Study will be conducted in a single urban area. The NICHD study of Early Child Care was conducted in several sites across the country, but is not nationally representative. In 1991, the follow-up of the National Maternal and Infant Health Survey obtained detailed information on the first three years of a birth cohort of children; however, there are no plans to continue this study.

Second, no study will permit *state-level measures*, which are becoming increasingly important as much of the policy focus shifts to the states.

Third, no survey proposes to collect *time-use data*. This is a critical need that no proposed effort will address.

Fourth, although surveys have incorporated the capacity to follow, interview, and assess Spanish-speaking students, no survey has the ability to assess and follow *Asian-language students* over time.

Fifth, the studies currently in the field are relatively small. A survey is needed with a large enough sample to be able to identify and follow *children with special needs and children not living with a parent.*

APPROACHES TO ADDRESSING DATA GAPS

There is no single ideal dataset. Different researchers have different purposes. Whereas some overlap is possible and desirable, the level of financing necessary is likely to preclude one dataset suiting everyone's needs. In addition, there is no such thing as unlimited resources; tradeoffs must be made, and the mission of the funding agency is always of prime concern. Consequently, the idea of multiple data collections appears desirable. Thus my first suggestion is to build on datasets already in existence by supplementing them with additional questions and assessments.

Supplement Ongoing Data Collections

Given the availability of 25 years of detailed information on families contained in it, supplementing the PSID would be my first priority. Preliminary estimates place the cost of a one-time data collection effort that includes age-appropriate child assessments at about $2.5 million. Collecting more limited data about children on a regular basis (a 8-minute supplement with questions asked of the parent) would cost on the order of $700,000 per year.

My second priority is to supplement the NLSY with more regular information on the mental health, criminal behavior, and drug and alcohol use of the child and parents. More information on fathers is needed on a regular basis. And it is important to make sure that the same questions are asked on every supplement. For example, many items were omitted from the 1990 survey because of funding problems; this produces gaps in the data and nightmares for analysts. A rough estimate of the cost of supplementing the NLSY in 1994 dollars is about $55,000 per minute for questions for all respondents. Asking questions of mothers only, such as about her child, would be about half this cost. Asking questions directly of children age 10 and older is considerably less expensive (perhaps one-quarter of the cost) because of the smaller sample size.

Given the enormous amount of information collected in the National Maternal and Infant Health Survey, my third priority is either to follow the National Maternal and Infant Health sample of children into their school years or to start a new cohort at birth; it could become a birth cohort study comparable to the British longitudinal study (Cherlin et al., 1991). One of the reasons another follow-back to the NMIHS has not been pursued is that the response rate in the first year was only 74 percent, although the follow-back response rate was 90 percent. Another 90 percent response rate would produce a total response rate of about 60 percent. Apparently some analysis was conducted and on that basis additional follow-back was rejected.[2] A new cohort that is smaller in size but followed for more years may be the cost-effective way to go.

Coordinate Existing Data Collection Efforts

Much more coordination and collaboration among institutions, so that there is at least some overlap between datasets, would allow more cross-study comparisons and validation than was previously possible. Asking several similar questions would be useful. For example, if the MECA study used the behavior problems index that is contained in the NLSY and compared the results in this shortened form with the results of other assessments, it would serve the field quite well; this type of cross-agency and disciplinary work would be very helpful. It would serve the NLSY well to include a high-quality diagnostic assessment of adults that has been used by NIMH regularly in its surveys. Regular assessment of substance abuse by parents in the NLSY would also be useful. Almost nothing is collected now on the mental health of mothers, which is a real omission, and there is only an occasional assessment of substance abuse. These measures could be obtained from NIMH, the National Institute on Drug Abuse, and the National Institute on Alcohol Abuse and Alcoholism. The four new surveys (mentioned in an earlier section) would do well to meet and discuss potential collaborations and cross-survey work.

Plan New Data Collections

National Survey of Children

A new survey of a representative sample of children of ages 0-17 is needed. Such a study would include a birth cohort and would permit analysis of all other age groups as well. The Census Bureau is interested in mounting such an effort, and its proposed Survey of Program Dynamics is a promising approach; however, I am not convinced that the planning and data collection of a new National Survey of Children should be a federal effort. Much of federal data collection does not allow enough planning time. In addition, a more flexible funding mechanism is needed—either a request for applications or a collaborative agreement with an agency. The model might be the Health and Retirement Survey, which is being conducted by a consortium of private institutions with funding from the National Institute on Aging. The Census Bureau could be one of the members of the consortium rather than the major actor. (The Census Bureau does not permit the release of information on neighborhoods, for example, and approval by the Office of Management and Budget is required.) A large chunk of such an effort could be conducted by the private sector with high response rates at considerable savings to the government.

A National Time-Use Survey of Children and Their Parents

Only one time-use study has been conducted, and results from this study are still being widely used (Carnegie Council, 1992). An entire survey should be conducted in this format. Given the trade-offs in other survey efforts, there is almost no possibility of conducting a modified time-use study along with other types of questions. The time-use portion must be central.

A ROLE FOR THE NATIONAL RESEARCH COUNCIL?

The final question I address is the possibility of a role for the National Research Council in examining/promoting more effective strategies for collecting and assembling national data on children and their families.

Disseminating the results of this workshop to all federal agencies and to the Office of Management and Budget is quite important. Agencies should be made aware that these interesting new studies are being planned. Although they may individually come to the attention of the Office of Management and Budget and/or Congress during the budget process, seeing them together as a package makes it easier to see overlaps and gaps.

In terms of promoting collaborative meetings, there is an immediate opportunity to get the relevant federal agencies together to discuss the four surveys currently being planned: the Program on Human Development and Criminal Behavior, the Multisite Study of Mental Health Services, the Early Childhood Longitudinal Study, and the Survey of Program Dynamics.

Another set of meetings could be held to discuss supplementing existing datasets, including the Michigan PSID, the NLSY mother-child sample, and the NMIHS. For a new National Survey of Children, there should be a collaborative effort originating from the field, rather a single agency effort. The first step might be a set of meetings with the interested agencies, researchers in the field, and funders. The second step would be to hold meetings with potential data collection firms, such as the National Opinion Research Center, WESTAT, the University of Michigan, and Temple University. It is extremely important to have the scientific community involved in and committed to the design and development of such a study from the beginning.

NOTES

1. An embedded substudy would interview a sample of Head Start children during the spring of the year before entering kindergarten.

2. The answer is not whether the response rate is low but whether the sample is in some way biased. Originally I recommended doing additional work to see whether the original sample is biased in a way that would reduce its value were it to continue to be followed. If it could be shown either to have minimal biases or if sampling weights could be constructed to reduce the known biases, then continuing to follow this cohort would be valuable. However, the statisticians do not agree with this and believe that a low response rate biases a survey, regardless of whether the responses are missing systematically or at random. The cost of one follow-up is on the order of $4 to 5 million, compared with the start-up cost of a new survey at an estimated $6-7 million.

REFERENCES

Baker, Paula C., Canada K. Keck, Frank L. Mott, and Stephen V. Quinlan
1993 *NLSY Child Handbook, Revised Edition.* Columbus, Ohio: Center for Human Resource Research, Ohio State University.

Beavers, W. Robert, and Robert Hampson
1992 Family Variables Related to Children's Capabilities and Interests in Education. Planning Paper for the National Center for Education Statistics Longitudinal Studies of Young Children. Southwest Family Institute.

Brick, Michael, Mary Collins, Carin Celebuski, Mary Jo Nolin, Theresa Squadere, Peter Ha, Jacqueline Wernimont, Jerry West, Kathryn Chandler, Elvie Hausken, and Jeffrey Owings
1992 *National Household Education Survey of 1991: Preprimary and Primary Data Files User's Manual.* Washington, D.C.: U.S. Department of Education.

Bumpass, Larry
1984 Children and marital disruption: a replication and update. *Demography* 21(February):71-82.

Bumpass, Larry, and James Sweet
1993 *Longitudinal Data on Families: The National Survey of Families and Households and the Design for the 5-year Reinterview.* Madison: The University of Wisconsin.

Carnegie Council on Adolescent Development
1992 *A Matter of Time: Risk and Opportunity in the Nonschool Hours.* New York: Carnegie Corporation.

Cherlin, A.J., F.F. Furstenberg, et al.
1991 Longitudinal studies of the effects of divorce on children in Great Britain and the United States. *Science* 252: 1386-1389.

Child Trends, Inc.
1993 *The JOBS Child Outcomes Study, Overview Briefing.* Washington, D.C.: Child Trends, Inc.

Copple, Carol, Sharon Deich, Lorelei Brush, and Sandra Hofferth
1993 *Learning Readiness: Promising Strategies.* Washington, D.C.: U.S. Department of Health and Human Services.

Duncan, G., J. Brooks-Gunn, and P. Klebanov
in press Economic deprivation and early childhood development. *Child Development.*

Earls, Felton
1993 *The Program on Human Development and Criminal Behavior: Executive Summary.* Washington, D.C.: National Institute of Justice.

Entwisle, Doris R.
1992 *Recommendations for the NCES Longitudinal Study of Early Childhood/Early Education.* Baltimore, Md.: Johns Hopkins University.

Espenshade, Thomas
1984 *Investing in Children: New Estimates of Parental Expenditures.* Washington, D.C.: The Urban Institute.

Fix, Michael and Wendy Zimmerman
1993 *Educating Immigrant Children: Chapter 1 in the Changing City.* Washington, D.C.: The Urban Institute Press.

Glantz, Frederic B., Judith Layzer, and Michael Battaglia
1988 *Study of the Child Care Food Program.* Cambridge, Mass.: Abt Associates.

Hofferth, Sandra
1985 Updating children's life course. *Journal of Marriage and the Family* 47:93-115.

Hofferth, Sandra, April Brayfield, Sharon Deich, and Pamela Holcomb
1991 *National Child Care Survey, 1990.* Washington, D.C.: The Urban Institute.

Hofferth, Sandra, Jerry West, Robin Henke, and Phillip Kaufman
1994 *Access to Preschool Programs among At-Risk Children.* Washington, D.C.: U.S. Department of Education.

Howes, Carollee
1992 Preschool Experiences. Paper prepared for the National Center for Educational Statistics. Los Angeles: University of California at Los Angeles.

Juster, F. Thomas, and Frank Stafford, eds.
1985 *Time, Goods, and Well-Being.* Ann Arbor: University of Michigan.

Karweit, Nancy
1992 *Elementary School and Classroom Characteristics Related to Student Preparation and Progress Through School.* Baltimore, Md.: Johns Hopkins University, Center for Social Organization of Schools.

Kellam, Sheppard
1993 School-Based Prevention Research on Early Risk Behaviors: Implications for Head Start and Beyond. Presented at the 2nd National Head Start Research Conference, Washington, D.C., November.

Kerckhoff, Alan C.
1992 Characteristics of Elementary Schools. Paper for the National Center for Education Statistics, Longitudinal Studies of Young Children, Duke University.

Kisker, Ellen, Sandra Hofferth, Deborah Phillips, and Elizabeth Farquhar
1991 *A Profile of Child Care Settings: Early Education and Care in 1990.* Washington, D.C.: U.S. Department of Education.

Korenman, Sanders, Jane Miller, and John Sjaastad
1994 Long-term Poverty and Child Development in the United States: Results from the NLSY. Minneapolis: University of Minnesota.

Kotelchuck, M., Schwartz, J., Anderka, K., and Finison, K.
1984 WIC participation and pregnancy outcomes: Massachusetts statewide evalution project. *American Journal of Public Health* 74(October):1086-1092.

Layzer, Jean I., Barbara D. Goodson, and Marc Moss
1993 *Life in Preschool: Volume One of an Observational Study of Early Childhood Programs for Disadvantaged Four-Year-Olds.* Cambridge, Mass.: Abt Associates.

Love, John M., Mary Ellin Logue, James V. Trudeau, and Katharine Thayer
1992 *Transitions to Kindergarten in American Schools.* Portsmouth, N.H.: RMC Research Corporation.

McLanahan, S.
1985 The reproduction of poverty. *American Journal of Sociology* 90:873-901.
1988 Family structure and dependency: early transitions to female household headship. *Demography* 25:1-16.

Moore, Kristin, and Nancy Snyder
1991 Cognitive attainment among firstborn children of adolescent mothers. *American Sociological Review* 56:612-624.

Mott, Frank L., and Elizabeth Menaghan
1993 Linkages betweeen Early Childhood Family Structure, Socioeconomic Well-Being and Middle-Childhood Socio-Emotional Development. Paper presented at the annual meeting of the Population Association of America, Cincinnati, April.

National Education Goals Panel
1993 *Reconsidering Children's Early Development and Learning: Toward Shared Beliefs and Vocabulary.* Draft Report. Washington, D.C.: National Education Goals Panel.

National Task Force on School Readiness
1991 *Caring Communities: Supporting Young Children and Families.* Alexandria, Va.: National Association of State Boards of Education.

Nettles, Saundra
1992 Community Structure and Social Support. A paper in support of planning activities for the NCES longitudinal survey of young children. Johns Hopkins University, Center for Social Organization of Schools.

NICHD Early Child Care Network
in press Child care and child development: The NICHD Study of Early Child Care. In S.L. Friedman and H.C. Haywood, eds., *Developmental Follow-up: Concepts, Domains and Methods.* New York: Academic Press.

O'Connell, Martin, and Amara Bachu
1992 Who's minding the kids? child care arrangements: fall 1988. *Current Population Reports* 30:70.

Office of the President
1994 *Budget of the United States Government.* Washington, D.C.: U.S. Government Printing Office.

Powell, Douglas R.
1992 Families and Young Children's School Readiness. Paper prepared for the National Center for Education Statistics. Department of Child Development and Family Studies, Purdue University.

Puma, Michael, Calvin Jones, Donald Rock, and Roberto Fernandez.
1993 *Prospects: The Congressionally Mandated Study of Educational Growth and Opportunity* (The Interim Report). Washington, D.C.: U.S. Department of Education.

Ramey, Craig, and Sharon L. Ramey
1992 Child and Family Transitions to School: Measuring Adaptation throughout the Elementary School Years. Paper prepared for the National Center for Education Statistics concerning the Longitudinal Studies Program of Young Children. Civitan International Research Center, University of Alabama at Birmingham.

Ramey, Sharon L., and Craig Ramey
in press Early educational intervention with disadvantaged children—to what effect? *Applied and Preventive Psychology.*

1993 *The National Head Start-Public School Early Childhood Transition Study: An Overview*. Birmingham, Ala.: Civitan International Research Center.

Schweinhart, Lawrence, Helen Barnes, and David Weikart
1993 *Significant Benefits: The High/Scope Perry Preschool Study through Age 27*. Ypsilanti, Mich: High/Scope Press.

Select Committee on Children, Youth, and Families
1985 *Opportunities for Success: Cost-Effective Programs for Children*. Washington, D.C.: U.S. Government Printing Office.

Seppanen, Patricia, John Love, Dianne Kaplan deVries, Lawrence Bernstein, Michelle Seligson, Fern Marx, and Ellen Kisker
1993 *National Study of Before- and After-School Programs*. Washington, D.C.: U.S. Department of Education.

Shonkoff, Jack
1992 The Conceptualization and Measurement of Child and Family Health. Paper prepared for the Longitudinal Studies Program of Young Children, University of Massachusetts.

Simpson, Gloria, David Keer, and Marcie Cynamon
1992 Plans for the 1993-94 National Health Interview Survey on Disability. Paper presented at the annual meeting of the American Statistical Association, August.

Stafford, Frank P.
1987 Women's work, sibling competition, and children's school performance. *American Economic Review* December: 972-980.

Timmer, Susan Goff, Jacquelynne Eccles, and Keith O'Brien
1985 How children use time. Pp. 353-382 in F. Thomas Juster and Frank Stafford, eds., *Time, Goods, and Well-Being*. Ann Arbor: University of Michigan.

West, Jerry
1992 Early Childhood Longitudinal Study (ECLS). Washington, D.C.: National Center for Education Statistics.

West, Jerry, Elvie Hausken, and Mary Collins
1993 *Profile of Preschool Children's Child Care and Early Education Program Participation*. Washington, D.C.: National Center for Educational Statistics.

Wolock, Isabel
1981 Child health and developmental problems and child maltreatment among AFDC families. *Journal of Sociology and Social Welfare* 8(1):83-96.

Woodward, Bob, and Benjamin Weiser
1994 Costs soar for children's disability program. *The Washington Post*, February 4.

Zill, Nicholas, Kristin A. Moore, Ellen Wolpow Smith, Thomas Stief, and Mary Jo Coiro
1995 The life circumstances and development of children in welfare families: a profile based on national data. In L. Chase-Lansdale and J. Brooks-Gunn, eds., *Escape from Poverty*. New York: Cambridge University Press.

Zill, Nicholas, and Margaret Daly, eds.
1993 *Researching the Family: A Guide to Survey and Statistical Data on U.S. Families*. Washington, D.C.: Child Trends, Inc.

Zill, Nicholas, and Charlotte Schoenborn
1990 Developmental, learning, and emotional problems: health of our nation's children, United States, 1988. *Advance Data* 190: November 16.

Federal Data on Educational Attainment and the Transition to Work

Aaron M. Pallas

Children and families have historically been viewed in the United States as matters of private, rather than public, concern. It has only been in the last two to three decades that the role of the state has expanded into issues of the health and well-being of families. Even today, however, most observers would be hard-pressed to argue that the United States has a national policy on children and families.

Nevertheless, as the interest of the state in the well-being of children and families has grown, the federal government has begun to debate and implement policies designed to promote the status of children and their families. These debates have often taken place in the absence of timely and accurate data on the well-being of children, and without the benefit of careful analysis of the implementation and effectiveness of the programs that have been serving children and families over the past 30 years. While it may be too harsh to claim that the lack of useful data has led to bad policy, there can be little question that timely, accurate, and relevant data on children and families have the capacity to inform public policy, particularly federal policies directed at the lives of children.

In this paper, I examine federal data on an important dimension of children's well-being: children's progress through school and into the labor force. A key challenge faced by all societies is the task of providing children with the personal qualities that enable them to become productive

Aaron M. Pallas is at the Department of Education, Michigan State University.

adult members of society. In our society, adulthood is often defined in terms of the ability of an individual to be financially and emotionally independent and self-sustaining, and is operationalized through the accession of adult work and family roles. Thus, moving into the labor force and forming a family through marriage or parenthood are key markers of adulthood.

Yet young people do not move into the labor force unassisted by social institutions. In industrial societies, schools are the social institutions charged with instilling the knowledge, skills, and values that will enable young people to become competent adults. Thus, policy concerns involving the productivity of the American labor force and the competitiveness of the United States in the world economy are frequently translated into concerns about the performance of the American education system. Most people still see a good education as the ticket to economic self-sufficiency, although there are competing explanations for why individuals who go farther through school are likely to achieve greater economic success than those who obtain less schooling.

I argue that the analysis of the ways in which American youth negotiate the transition to adulthood reflects an important tension between individual trajectories and the role of social institutions. Institutionally based data often are not reflective of the set of pathways that individuals travel as they become adults. Conversely, studies of individuals independent of the organizational and institutional contexts in which they are situated may not reveal the important role that schools and employers play in structuring educational attainment and the transition into the labor force. I suggest, therefore, a need for a set of data collection mechanisms that balance data on individuals and on institutions.

THE DEMAND FOR INFORMATION ON EDUCATIONAL ATTAINMENT AND THE TRANSITION INTO THE LABOR FORCE

In this section I briefly review some of the major policy questions posed at the federal level that concern educational attainment and the transition into the labor force. These questions have taken on a heightened importance in recent years, in the context of rising concerns about the performance of the education system and its capacity to prepare young people for productive work roles in society, and about the apparent decline of U.S. competitiveness in the world economy. It is widely believed that a better-educated cadre of youth—both with respect to the quantity and quality of the education they receive—is the key to regaining the economic growth and productivity that characterized the post-World War II economy.

I further subdivide the relevant policy questions into two categories: descriptive and analytic. Descriptive questions inquire about the nature and scope of a policy domain and are intended to gauge basic information about its current status and trends. Such questions are often addressed with social indicator data that provide coarse but useful information about the status and direction of change in a system. "What is the youth unemployment rate this month?" is an example of a descriptive policy question, and the seasonally adjusted monthly unemployment rate for youth ages 16-24 is an example of the data that might be used to address this question.

Analytic policy questions typically inquire about the relations among variables. Such questions are often used to inform decisions about policy implementation and its likely effects. The questions are frequently posed in cause-and-effect terms and typically are narrower in their scope than descriptive policy questions. "Does participation in a training program for out-of-school youth decrease youth unemployment?" is an example of an analytic policy question, and a carefully controlled study comparing the unemployment rates of program participants and similar nonparticipants is an example of the data that might be used to address this question.

Educational Attainment

I begin by examining some of the key policy questions regarding educational attainment. In the U.S. schooling system, primary schooling is universal, and virtually all young people attend secondary schools, although not all complete their secondary education. Policy makers are frequently concerned with the key branching points of high school completion, postsecondary access, and postsecondary completion.

Descriptive Policy Questions

Since high school completion is widely regarded as a minimum prerequisite for the development of the skills, knowledge, and values needed to succeed in the emerging economy, there is a great deal of interest in understanding who is graduating from high school and who is not. The overall high school dropout and completion rates are important indicators of the health of the education system, although these rates have been measured in many different ways, often leading to widely divergent estimates of the scope of the problem. Moreover, given the nation's historic commitment to equality of opportunity, coupled with concerns about an emerging underclass, policy makers wish to know whether dropout and completion rates differ for traditionally disadvantaged populations, such as racial and ethnic minorities, women, and the poor, or for residents of central cities or recent immigrants to the United States. There also is interest in whether dropout and completion rates vary across different regions of the country, and in the timing of dropping out in the secondary school career: Do dropout rates differ by students' age or grade level?

Several of these questions have been codified in the National Education Goals agreed to by President Bush and the 50 governors in 1989. Goal 2 states: "By the year 2000, the high school graduation rate will increase to at least 90 percent." The two additional objectives associated with Goal 2 state: "The nation must dramatically reduce its dropout rate, and 75 percent of those students who do drop out will successfully complete a high school degree or its equivalent" and "The gap in high school graduation rates between American students from minority backgrounds and their non-minority counterparts will be eliminated."

Although the National Education Goals are surprisingly silent on participation in postsecondary schooling, there nevertheless are a host of long-standing descriptive policy concerns about access to and completion of postsecondary schooling. This is particularly true in light of the longstanding federal role in financing higher education. It is estimated that more than a third of all undergraduates in recent years have received some form of federal financial aid for their postsecondary schooling. Many of the same descriptive questions about high school completion are replicated at the postsecondary level. Policy makers are interested in knowing whether enrollment in and completion of postsecondary schooling varies according to the social characteristics of youth, including their gender, racial/ethnic identity, family income level, and age. Moreover, in light of the differentiation of the American higher education system, there is great interest in variability in the type of institutions and programs in which students enroll, particularly the contrasts between two-year and four-year postsecondary institutions and between academic and nonacademic programs of study. In some instances, in which a particular postsecondary program is strongly linked to a particular career trajectory, policy makers may wish to know the number and types of students enrolling in particular programs, such as those leading to careers in science and engineering, or mathematics and science teaching, for example.

Some of these descriptive questions at the secondary and postsecondary levels may be addressed through both surveys of individuals and surveys of institutions. Basic enrollment data, for example, are produced by the National Center for Education Statistics' annual Common Core of Data (CCD) program at the elementary-secondary level and the Integrated Postsecondary Education Data System (IPEDS) program at the postsecondary level. However, such institutional data collections have limited utility for many of the analytic issues considered below.

Analytic Policy Questions

At the secondary level, the key analytic policy questions take two forms. The first might be called "basic" policy research, in the sense that the goal is to provide a greater understanding of the school dropout phenomenon that might be used to generate potential policy instruments designed to promote high school completion. The second might be labeled "applied" policy research, in the sense that it pertains to understanding the impact of already formulated programs and policies on school completion.

The basic analytic policy concerns at the secondary level consist of a set of questions about the causes and consequences of dropping out of high school, including the dynamics of school enrollment. We still know rather little about why young people leave school before completion, and what happens to them after they do so. We also have relatively little insight into why individuals travel different pathways to high school completion (i.e., regular day high school diplomas, General Educational Development or GED credentials, and other high school completion credentials), why they travel these pathways on different timetables (i.e., moving in and out of the education system), or what the socioeconomic consequences of these different pathways might be.

The concerns I have identified here parallel those raised in a recent report from the Office of Educational Research and Improvement on reaching the high school completion goal of the National Education Goals (OERI Goal 2 Work Group, 1994). That report suggested four questions that the authors believed warranted further research that might inform efforts to make progress toward the goal: (1) What do we know about mainstream dropouts? How can we explain the large numbers of youngsters who, without seeming disadvantaged, still fail to complete high school? Conversely, why do so many more of their peers succeed in completing high school? (2) What are the factors that lead Hispanics, American Indians, and students with disabilities to leave school at greater rates than those in the mainstream? (3) What are the consequences of completing a GED rather than a regular high school diploma? (4) To what extent does the lure of adolescent employment and the challenge of teenage parenting influence the prospects for higher graduation rates?

The applied analytic policy concerns at the secondary level pertain primarily to the evaluation of specific policies and programs designed to influence the high school graduation rate, and in addition to understanding the *unanticipated* consequences of other educational and social programs for the high school graduation rate. For example, the focus of the school reform movement of the 1980s was the attempt to raise standards for student performance—by increasing high school graduation requirements, implementing high-stakes exit tests, and increasing student workloads. Although policy makers may not have intended such reforms to have an adverse effect on school dropout rates, in the absence of new resources targeted to help marginal students achieve the new standards, it seems likely that these reforms might have had an unintended effect on school completion. Yet we have little concrete evidence of the impact of the school reform movement on the likelihood of school completion. Nor do we have definitive evidence on the consequences of incentive programs that rely on rewards or sanctions to spur students to stay in school, such as those that promise college tuition money to youth who complete high school, those that deny driver's licenses to individuals who leave school before graduation, and those that lower welfare benefits to the families of youth who stop going to school.

There also are naturally occurring variations in the school experiences and environments of children and youth that may be consequential for their chances of staying in school. Classroom reward and evaluation systems, the organization of instruction into homogeneous ability groups and age-graded classrooms, grade retention policies, school size, and curricula all represent factors at least partly amenable to policy manipulation that might have consequences for whether young people complete their high school educations.

At the postsecondary level, the central analytic questions concern the intertwining of families, work, and postsecondary schooling. There is considerable interest in the ways in which families contribute to the financing of the postsecondary schooling of dependent children, and in the ways in which independent youth finance their college educations. Since the federal government is a significant source of financial aid for many young college attendees, policy makers wish to know the consequences for postsecondary enrollment and persistence of variations in the levels and sources of federal and other financial aid to students, and of changes in the eligibility criteria for aid programs. It is, moreover, important to understand postsecondary schooling in the context of other social institutions in which youth participate, such as work, family, and the military, to name some of the most important ones. Increasing numbers of youth are combining work and postsecondary schooling, and many choose between military service and postsecondary schooling upon graduating from high school. The social and economic consequences of variations in the timing of postsecondary schooling, and the ways in which it is sequenced with family, work, and military experiences, are not well understood.

Transition into the Labor Force

Unlike that for educational attainment, our knowledge about school-to-work transitions is extremely limited. We lack powerful theories of how young people negotiate the transition from school to work and what social forces are important in that transition. In the absence of strong theories, it is unlikely that existing federal data sources will be especially helpful in illuminating the most pressing policy concerns. Such data are grounded in an understanding of the youth labor market and of learning in school and on the job that is rapidly being superseded by more complex views.

For example, human capital theories have viewed skill or ability as the centerpiece of labor markets, with individuals selling their skills and employers purchasing them. In this view, skill supply and demand is among the most important policy considerations in the transition into the labor force. But this view takes skill or ability as a relatively fixed feature of individuals *independent of their learning contexts*, and thus assumes that the skill, ability, and learning demonstrated in school can readily transfer to the workplace. The cognitive demands of the workplace, and the ways in which it facilitates or inhibits ongoing learning, are left largely unexamined. If, however, one adopts a constructivist view of learning that sees the construction of knowledge as inextricably linked to the learning environment, then it would not make sense to view the school-to-work transition as a simple matter of transferring those cognitive skills acquired or developed in school to the workplace. Rather, the transition is much more complicated, as each setting for learning reshapes what individuals know and are able to apply in the next setting. Moreover, as individuals change and develop over time, so too do workplace learning environments, which implies a need to build a dynamic conception of work settings into research designs. Even those data collections that do in fact assess aspects of the workplace typically conceive of it as static, rather than changing. This is especially problematic under conditions of rapid technological change, which clearly characterizes a number of industries in the United States. Such technological change can result in either increased *or* lessened cognitive demands on young workers, depending on the industry or technology in question. Our data collection mechanisms need to take account of the impact of such change on the nature of youth employment.

These are not the only such alternative perspectives on the transition to work, and it would be taking this paper far afield to explore even these approaches in greater detail. But the existence of such competing ways of conceptualizing the problem—or, more precisely, the lack of *any* adequate way of conceptualizing the problem at this time—points out the limits of available data collections to inform our understanding of the transition to work. This understanding seems more likely to emerge from rich field studies than from federal statistics-gathering efforts.

Descriptive Policy Questions

Perhaps the most basic descriptive policy questions regarding the transition into the labor force pertain to the quantity and quality of youth employment. Policy makers are interested in the incidence and intensity of employment and unemployment among youth, both during and after periods in which they are enrolled in school. Among those youth who are employed, the number of hours worked, type of work, and wages all are fundamental features of the youth employment picture. Moreover, policy makers want to know how youth employment and unemployment vary by the social background of youth, including their race/ethnicity, gender, household composition, family income level, geographic location, age, and educational attainment, and whether these patterns are stable or changing over time.

All of these factors are measurable. Unfortunately, perhaps the most important descriptive policy questions are not as easily operationalized. For example, from the standpoint of human capital theory, the key to understanding the youth labor market and the policy issues surrounding it is the supply of and demand for skill. Youth bring with them to a job a set of skills derived from schooling, previous work experience, and family and community influences. Conversely, employers seek employees with the requisite skills to carry out the tasks required of workers in their firms. The match—or mismatch—between the supply of and demand for skill has more profound implications for youth labor market policy than virtually any other feature. Yet the little direct evidence on skill supply and demand among youth does not derive from large-scale federal statistical surveys, but rather from small, industry-specific or firm-specific case studies. Even individual industries or firms, however, are not homogeneous or highly stable over time, so that generalizations are extremely difficult.

Analytic Policy Questions

Many of the important analytic policy questions regarding the transition to work view the youth labor market in the context of its connections to other social institutions, particularly schooling, families, and communities. Thus, attention is directed to what might be called the school-to-work transition system, or the "linkage" system joining schooling and the economy. Whereas the match or mismatch in skill supply and demand is the most important feature of the linkage system, there are other important policy issues to be explored as well. For example, how do schools help young people make the transition from school to work, and how might they be more successful? How do partnerships or contracts between schools and employers affect the ways in which youth negotiate the transition from school to work? What kinds of signals do schools provide to employers about the qualities of youthful workers, and how can we improve the quality of information available to both youth and employers about each other (see Rosenbaum et al., 1990)?

Another set of policy questions is concerned with the linkages between work and families and communities. Mizell (1988) identifies a pressing need to understand how families and communities influence adolescent work behavior. The transition to work often is viewed in the context of specific communities, because the youth labor market is not a national market, but rather a local one. Thus, local community conditions—e.g., the kinds of social dislocations defined by weakened social institutions that William Julius Wilson has written about in *The Truly Disadvantaged* (1987)—frame youth attitudes toward work, the reasons why youth work, and the opportunities youth have for productive work.

Other policy questions focus on the characteristics of the jobs in which youth work more so than on the individuals working in those jobs. For example, what kinds of opportunities for advancement, training and learning are offered in the workplaces where youth are found? In what ways do workplaces function as learning environments for youth, and how is this learning connected to future success in adult work and social life (Rosenbaum et al., 1990)?

The kinds of analytic policy questions I have described here are difficult ones to address, and we may not currently have the tools to shed light on all or even many of them. In some cases, we may be able to learn a great deal simply by piggybacking some new survey items on existing data collections, thereby preserving existing data while forging a new link to additional questions of interest. But not all instances will be this easy. Some questions are not easily approached via sample surveys. Questions about learning in the workplace, for example, may be as resistant to paper-and-pencil measures as questions about learning in school. Still other questions may require detailed observation or understanding of work sites or data from employers. In either event, samples of individuals separated from the organizational context of their work experience may not be the best means for understanding some of these complex questions.

There are, to be sure, other kinds of questions for which surveys of individuals may be appropriate. For example, although earlier studies have addressed issues such as the consequences of adolescent work experience, the connections between school performance and getting a good job, and the ways in which adolescent work before school-leaving is connected to work after leaving school, such studies need to be updated. In some cases, the data on which they are based are now quite old, and there is no guarantee that they apply equally well to the tighter labor market conditions that confront the current generation of youth. General-purpose longitudinal surveys of individuals have been the primary means for addressing the kinds of issues I am describing, and they will probably continue to be so in the future.

Charner and Fraser (1988), in reflecting on the kinds of policy issues noted above, call for an integrated database focused on youth employment (p.55):

> Currently there does not exist a single data base which examines the detailed patterns of student participation in work experiences; the multiple dimensions of the nature of these work experiences; the roles and responsibilities of students as workers; and the effects of differential work experiences on different educational, family, social, and personal short and long-term outcomes. Such a dataset on a representative sample of students from different subgroups of the population is clearly needed.

They go on to attempt to specify some of the requisite data elements in such a data base (p.56):

> A set of common questions needs to be developed which can be used by future researchers. These questions need to cover, at a minimum, the following: (a) work histories including: type of job, duration, hours worked, wages, length of employment, employer, and benefits; (b) multiple dimensions of work including: occupational self direction, position in the organizational structure, job pressures, and extrinsic risks and rewards; (c) reasons for working including: financial, experiential, learning, and social-psychological reasons; and (d) outcomes including: attitudinal and behavioral outcomes, both short and long-term.

Charner and Fraser's (1988) data collection agenda is ambitious, but it does point out some of the gaps in the existing data on the transition to work. It is to these data, and the statistical programs that produce them, that I now turn.

THE AVAILABLE FEDERAL STATISTICAL DATA SOURCES

In this section, I describe the key federal sources of data on educational attainment and the transition into the labor force. I include in this description major data collection activities carried out by or sponsored by federal government agencies, such as the Census Bureau's Current Population Survey and the Longitudinal Studies Program of the National Center for Education Statistics (NCES). I also consider the Panel Study of Income Dynamics (PSID), an important ongoing study that originated in the Office of Economic Opportunity and is now funded through the National Science Foundation and various private sources. Because it is no longer sponsored by the federal government, perhaps it is inaccurate to describe the PSID as a federal data source. Nevertheless, I include it because of its unique properties and the capacity of the study to address important questions pertaining to schooling, work, and the life course. A brief summary of these datasets and their pertinent features is displayed in Table 1.

Current Population Survey

The Current Population Survey (CPS) is a sample survey conducted by the Bureau of the Census in the Department of Commerce, with the collaboration of the Bureau of Labor Statistics in the Department of Labor. Over its 53-year history it has been the primary source for perhaps the most prominent indicator of the health of the American economy, the seasonally adjusted monthly unemployment rate. The CPS also produces data on the characteristics of the labor force, including the number and characteristics of individuals who are employed, unemployed, or not in the labor force. The survey provides basic data on the labor force participation of individuals, including their earnings, numbers of hours worked, occupations and industrial classifications, and job search strategies (among the unemployed), as well as basic demographic data on households. In addition, there are periodic supplements sponsored by the Bureau of the Census or other federal agencies that provide additional information on such topics as school enrollment and child care.

The CPS samples approximately 60,000 households drawn from over 700 areas (typically counties and independent cities) located across the 50 states and the District of Columbia. The sampled households are rotated, with each household in the sample for four consecutive months, then out of the sample for eight additional months, and then back in the sample for four consecutive months. This design is intended to reduce sampling errors in month-to-month or year-to-year comparisons by ensuring a certain amount of overlap in the sample composition over short time periods (Bureau of Labor Statistics, 1988). Although the CPS data are longitudinal, the 16-month span of a household's participation in the sample is much more like a snapshot than a moving picture of the school-to-work transition. A household informant provides data on the civilian noninstitutionalized household members age 16 or over, totaling approximately 113,000 individuals each month (Bureau of Labor Statistics, 1988). The CPS sample thus generalizes to the civilian noninstitutionalized population of the United States age 16 years of age or over.

The CPS has recently undergone extensive revisions to its survey instrument and data collection procedures. The questionnaire has been revised to clarify existing definitions, incorporate changes in definitions recommended by several commissions and advisory groups, and improve the wording and sequencing of questions. In addition, all interviews are now carried out with the aid of computers, enabling the use of dependent interviewing (using information from the previous month's interview in the cur-

TABLE 1 Summary of Federal Statistical Data on Educational Attainment and the Transition to Work

Study Title	Sample	Periodicity	Data Sources	Key Measures
Current Population Survey (CPS)	Rotating nationally representative sample of 60,000 households	Monthly — households are in sample for 4 months, then out of sample for 8 months, then back in sample for 4 months	Household informant interview provides data on civilian noninstitutionalized household members age 16 orover	Labor force participation; school enrollment; educational attainment; income and earnings; basic demographic data
National Longitudinal Study of the High School Class of 1972 (NLS-72)	Nationally representative sample of high school seniors in 1972 — sample ranges from 17,000 students in base year to 12,000 students in fifth follow-up	Base-year survey in 1972, with follow-up surveys in 1973, 1974, 1976, 1979 and 1986	Student questionnaires; base year standardized test battery; school records from respondents' high schools; postsecondary transcripts	Family background; educational and occupational plans; postsecondary schooling, work and military experience; attitudes and values
High School and Beyond (HS&B)	Nationally representative sample of 30,000 high school sophomores and 28,000 high school seniors enrolled in more than 1,000 public and private schools in 1980	Base-year survey in 1980; follow-up surveys for both cohorts in 1982, 1984, and 1986; follow-up survey for sophomore cohort in 1992	Student questionnaires; cognitive test battery in base year and first follow-up; base-year parent and teacher questionnaires; high school administrator and teacher survey; postsecondary education transcripts	Family background; school experiences; educational and occupational plans; work experience; postsecondary schooling; attitudes and values; family formation

continued on next page

TABLE 1 Continued

Study Title	Sample	Periodicity	Data Sources	Key Measures
National Education Longitudinal Study of 1988 (NELS:88)	Nationally representative sample of 25,000 eighth graders enrolled in more than 1,000 public and private schools in 1988	Base-year survey in 1988; follow-up surveys in 1990, 1992, and 1994; scheduled follow-up) in 1996, with possibility of one or two additional follow-ups at two-year intervals	Student questionnaires; cognitive test battery in base year and first and second follow-ups; parent questionnaire in base year and second follow-up; school questionnaires; teacher questionnaires; dropout questionnaires	Family background; language use; school experiences; work experiences; plans for the future; parental involvement; teachers' perceptions; school policies and practices; curriculum content
Beginning Postsecondary Study (BPS)	Nationally representative sample of 7,000 students entering postsecondary schooling in 1989-90	Base-year survey in 1989-90; follow-up survey in 1992; scheduled follow-ups at two-year intervals	Student questionnaires; National Postsecondary Student Aid Study (NPSAS:90) parent questionnaires; postsecondary transcripts	Family background and financial data; postsecondary schooling and employment experiences, including academic progress, field of study, persistence, and future plans; family formation; financial aid and expenses associated with postsecondary schooling
Baccalaureate and Beyond Study (B&B)	Nationally representative sample of 16,000 students completing their baccalaureate degrees in 1992-93	Base-year survey in 1992-93; scheduled follow-ups at 1, 3, 6, 9, and 12-year intervals	National Postsecondary Student Aid Study (NPSAS) student and parent questionnaires; institutionally generated student records	Family background; financing of undergraduate and graduate education; educational experiences in undergraduate and graduate school; employment experience; family formation; future expectations

National Longitudinal Study of Youth (NLSY)	Nationally representative sample of 12,000 noninstitutionalized civilian and military youth ages 14 to 21 in 1979	Base-year survey in 1979; annual reinterviews	Respondent interviews; high school transcripts; Armed Services Vocational Aptitude Battery scores; assessments of children of mothers in the sample .	Sources of income; training; employment and unemployment spells; occupational mobility; attitudes about and knowledge of work; education; family formation; child care; child cognitive and socioemotional development
Panel Study of Income Dynamics (PSID)	National sample of approximately 8,000 households, beginning in 1968	Base-year interview in 1968; annual reinterviews	Respondent interviews	Sources of income; employment and earnings histories; family composition; household expenditures; housing; child care information; disability and illness; job search strategies; retirement plans and experience; savings patterns; standardized test performance

rent interview) and reducing errors produced by complicated skip patterns (Polivka and Rothgeb, 1993).

Of special interest here is the revision of the question eliciting educational attainment in the CPS. Beginning in January 1992, the CPS item asks, "What is the highest level of school . . . has completed or the highest degree . . . has received?" The response options include:

> "less than 1st grade,"
> "1st, 2nd, 3rd, or 4th grade,"
> "5th or 6th grade,"
> "7th or 8th grade,"
> "9th grade,"
> "10th grade,"
> "11th grade,"
> "12th grade NO DIPLOMA,"
> "HIGH SCHOOL GRADUATE—high school DIPLOMA, or the equivalent (for example: GED),"
> "Some college but no degree,"
> "Associate degree in college—Occupational/vocational program,"
> "Associate degree in college—academic program,"
> "Bachelor's degree (For example: BA, AB, BS),"
> "Master's degree (For example: MA, MS, MEng, MEd, MSW, MBA),"
> "Professional School Degree (For example: MD, DDS, DVM, LLB, JD)," and
> "Doctorate degree (For example: PhD, EdD)."

I belabor this because this new item is a substantial improvement over the old item, which for more than 40 years consisted of two parts: "What is the highest grade or year of regular school . . . has ever attended?" and "Did . . . complete the grade?" As Kominski and Siegel (1993) note, the old item did not identify specific degrees, so that analysts were obliged to infer attainment of a degree from years of schooling. This was a particular problem in the classification of high school graduates, as some individuals have completed 12 years of school without obtaining a high school diploma, while others have completed fewer than 12 years of school but obtained a credential equivalent to a high school diploma such as a GED or an alternative credential. Although the change in this item does interrupt a time series spanning 50 years, Kominski and Siegel (1993) argue persuasively that the meaning of educational attainment had changed sufficiently over this period to make the old item misleading.

The CPS data also are used to provide estimates of the national high school dropout rate. Because the October school enrollment supplement asks about both current enrollment status and enrollment status one year prior to the survey date, as well as current attainment level, it is possible to identify those individuals who were enrolled in grades 10-12 a year ago, are not currently enrolled in grades 10-12, and have not completed high school (Kominski, 1990). Such individuals may be said to have dropped out of school in the past year. NCES, using the October CPS data, reports the proportion of such individuals in a particular population group as the *event* dropout rate (see, e.g., Kaufman et al., 1992).

NCES also relies on the October CPS to estimate the proportion of a particular population group that has not completed high school and is not currently enrolled in school. This proportion is referred to as the *status* dropout rate, because it estimates the proportion of a population group that has the status of dropout at a particular point in time.

The primary strengths of the CPS for policy purposes are its periodicity and ability to generate national estimates. The data can be used to generate annual trends in the educational and occupational attainments of the U.S. young adult population, including rates of secondary and postsecondary access and degree completion and of employment and unemployment. Subject to variations in question wording and survey procedures, the CPS data provide a consistent data series for broad trends in the schooling and work accomplishments of youth.

The CPS data are not as useful for addressing policy concerns targeted at specific subpopulations, such as minority youth. Because the numbers of minorities enrolled in grades 10-12 in the CPS sample in a given year is not large, estimates of statistics pertaining to them (e.g., the dropout rate for Hispanic males) are subject to substantial sampling errors. This problem is, of course, heightened if the subpopulation is further subdivided by level of last grade attended or income level. Kominski (1990) used 3-year moving averages to estimate such rates. Such moving averages increase the sample size for a particular statistic, thereby reducing the sampling variability, but simultaneously increase the nonsampling errors by relying on data from different years.

Hauser (1991:9) notes several other difficulties in using the CPS data as a backdrop to policy formulation.

> There are some problems in using the CPS data to measure adolescent educational transitions. The samples become excessively small and statistically unreliable when we try to focus on key transitions, especially among minority groups. Family income is not measured well, and academic ability is not measured at all. . . . We lose the link with parents when children leave their parents' household and do not live in group quarters at school. The CPS does not cover persons in the military or in institutions, like prisons and jails, that now house a substantial minority of young adults. The CPS tells us little about the schools or colleges in which students are enrolled; we learn only whether enrollment is at a 2-year or 4-year public

> or private institution. Other recent content changes have reduced the usefulness of the October data. . . . At the same time, unlike the institutional or longitudinal surveys of NCES, the October CPS does provide annual data on college entry and enrollment.

In sum, then, the CPS functions best as a relatively crude indicator of trends in the educational attainment and employment experiences of youth. It is of less value for policy issues that demand greater detail in the descriptions of the schooling or employment experiences of youth, and of limited use for examining the dynamics of schooling and the transition to work.

It is hard to imagine major changes to the structure of the CPS. Its primary purpose as a barometer of the health of the economy is so important that any change that might jeopardize the reliability and validity of the data series is likely to meet with stiff resistance. Even seemingly small changes to the structure of the CPS—for example, oversampling minorities or the poor—could have adverse effects on estimates of key educational and economic trends. More fundamental changes in the study design—more detailed questions regarding schooling and work, or an extended follow-up, to cite but a few examples—seem out of the question, due to the technical problems and costs that might ensue. There are some small changes, coming on the heels of the recent CPS redesign, that might be undertaken, but the CPS is unlikely to be transformed in ways that would fundamentally alter its use for monitoring educational attainment and the transition to adulthood.

The next set of federal data collections complement the strengths and weaknesses of the CPS. Whereas the periodicity and stability of the CPS allows for a timely, consistent measure of trends in the educational attainment and employment of youth, the National Longitudinal Studies Program of NCES examines cohorts spaced 8 to 10 years apart. However, this latter program provides much greater analytic detail on the dynamics of educational attainment and employment than is provided by the CPS.

The NCES National Longitudinal Studies Program

For more than two decades, NCES has been conducting longitudinal studies of large, nationally representative samples of school-age youth. The National Longitudinal Studies Program has been an important resource for the analysis of students' experiences as they move through secondary school and into early adulthood. The program has become even more valuable in recent years, through NCES' outreach and dissemination efforts. Although the datasets were once extremely cumbersome to work with, they now are much more accessible and user-friendly, and NCES is more directly involved in the training of new users. The datasets are so rich that the hundreds of doctoral dissertations, journal articles and books based on them merely scratch the surface of their potential contributions to our understanding of schooling and the transition to adulthood. When Ellis Page, describing the initial analyses of the base year of High School and Beyond in 1981, said, "Welcome to the data feast!" he was not exaggerating.

NCES has fielded three national longitudinal studies of secondary students that have traced their educational and occupational careers into young adulthood: the National Longitudinal Study of the High School Class of 1972 (1972), High School and Beyond (HS&B), and the National Education Longitudinal Study of 1988 (NELS:88). In addition, NCES is currently planning a new study in this series, the National Education Longitudinal Study of 1998 (NELS:98), that will begin with a new cohort of middle or high-school-age students in 1998 (Davis and Sonnenberg, 1993). NCES has also begun two longitudinal studies focusing on participation in postsecondary education: the Beginning Postsecondary Student Longitudinal Study (BPS), and the Baccalaureate and Beyond Longitudinal Study (B&B). Each of these studies is discussed below.

The National Longitudinal Study of the High School Class of 1972

The National Longitudinal Study of the High School Class of 1972 (NLS-72) is a stratified probability sample of public and private high school students enrolled in the 12th grade in spring 1972. The sample design called for surveying 18 high school seniors in more than 1,000 high schools across the country. Schools in low-income areas and with high minority enrollments were oversampled. There have been five follow-up surveys, in 1973, 1974, 1976, 1979, and 1986. The NLS-72 study thus follows a single cohort of youth from (approximately) age 18 to age 32. The sample size increased from approximately 17,000 students in the base year to approximately 21,000 students in the first follow-up, due to the addition of base-year nonrespondents. Response rates for the follow-up surveys are uniformly high. The 1986 follow-up, a subsample of the original sample, included more than 12,000 individuals.

In each wave of the NLS-72 study, respondents completed an approximately hour-long survey questionnaire tapping aspects of family background, educational and occupational plans and experiences, and attitudes and values. The follow-up questionnaires, collected primarily through the mail, typically focused on respondents' experiences since the preceding follow-up. In the base year, respondents also completed a standardized test battery. A subset of the sample completed a standardized test in the 1979 follow-up. In addition, NCES gathered school record information from the respondents' high schools and conducted a Postsecondary Education Transcript Study in 1984.

The NLS-72 study is limited in its capacity to inform our understanding of the contribution of secondary schools to the educational and occupational careers of youth. Since the survey began with students enrolled in the 12th grade in spring 1972, there are only a small number of students who did not complete high school, even though about one-sixth of all 18- to 19-year-olds (and a substantially higher number of minority youth) in 1972 were neither enrolled in school nor high school graduates. The survey provides no information whatsoever on the experiences of this group, which might have experienced the most difficulty in the transition to adulthood. Moreover, the formative educational and social experiences of these youth are addressed either retrospectively or, more commonly, not at all. Because there are no data on students' achievements or attitudes that predate the 1972 base-year data collection, it is virtually impossible to examine the contribution of schools and schooling to the educational and occupational trajectories these youth traveled.

The High School and Beyond Study

NCES began the High School and Beyond (HS&B) study in 1980. Once again, the design called for a two-stage stratified national probability sample of high school students, with schools the first-stage sampling unit and students within schools the second-stage unit. The study randomly selected approximately 1,100 public and private high schools across the country, oversampling high-achieving private schools, public schools with concentrations of Hispanic students, Catholic schools with large proportions of minority students, and alternative public schools. Up to 36 sophomores and 36 seniors were sampled within each of these schools, yielding a base-year sample size of approximately 30,000 high school seniors (the HS&B senior cohort) and 28,000 high school sophomores (the HS&B sophomore cohort). A total of 12,000 members of the senior cohort were followed up in 1982, 1984, and 1986; roughly 27,000 members of the sophomore cohort were followed up in 1982, and about 15,000 members were followed up in 1984, 1986, and 1992. The senior cohort thus has been followed from approximately age 18 to age 24, whereas the sophomore cohort has been followed from approximately age 16 to age 28. The HS&B study was designed to facilitate comparisons with NLS-72, and in fact there have been a series of analytic studies comparing the experiences of both the sophomore cohort and the senior cohort with the cohort of high school seniors in NLS-72 (see, e.g., Ekstrom et al., 1988; Alexander et al., 1987).

In the base year of the study, members of both cohorts completed an hour-long questionnaire and a cognitive test battery of similar length. In addition, a school administrator filled out a school questionnaire, and a subsample of parents of sample members completed a parent questionnaire. A teacher of the sampled student filled out a brief comment checklist on the student's habits and performance. As with the NLS-72 base-year student questionnaire, the HS&B base-year student questionnaire emphasized family background, school experiences, and future educational and occupational plans, including financial planning for college. Subsequent follow-up questionnaires elicited detailed information on the characteristics of jobs held and postsecondary schooling, as well as attitudes, values, and family formation. Spells of schooling, work, marriage, and childbearing are noted via start and stop dates for each event, thus providing relatively complete event histories over the period of time covered by the follow-ups. The first follow-up also administered the cognitive test battery to the sophomore cohort.

Of special interest is the first follow-up of the sophomore cohort, due to the window it provided on dropping out of high school. Because the HS&B study surveyed (and even administered a cognitive test battery to) youth identified as out of school at the time of the first follow-up, it has provided very useful information on the causes and consequences of dropping out of high school and on the dynamics of high school completion.

There have been a number of supplemental data collections carried out under the auspices of HS&B, including the Postsecondary Education Transcript Study of the senior cohort in 1984 and a similar study of the sophomore cohort scheduled for 1993 (Davis and Sonnenberg, 1993). Perhaps the most prominent is the Administrator and Teacher Survey carried out in 1984. Historically, NCES surveys have been more attuned to individual attainments and career trajectories than to the influence of organizational environments on those attainments. Hence, the questionnaires are rarely designed to assess the influence of educational programs and policies on student outcomes. In light of this, a consortium of educational research and development centers returned to about 500 of the original 1,100 high schools in the base year of the HS&B study in 1984 to gather additional information on topics such as school climate, governance, and school improvement programs. Surveying one administrator and up to 30 teachers in each of these schools, the consortium generated a dataset that could be linked to the HS&B student data to provide reliable information on school organization. Unfortunately, the assumptions needed to use 1984 data on school organization to inform an understanding of students' experiences between 1980 and 1982 are not always plausible (see, e.g., Chubb and Moe, 1990).

The National Education Longitudinal Study of 1988

The National Education Longitudinal Study of 1988 (NELS:88) was the third NCES longitudinal study, and its design retained many of the features of NLS-72 and HS&B and added to them. The most important design change was a shift in the grade cohort followed over time. Whereas NLS-

72 traced high school seniors, and HS&B had both a sophomore cohort and a senior cohort, the NELS:88 study began with a cohort of students enrolled in the 8th grade in spring 1988. As with NLS-72 and HS&B, the design specified a two-stage probability sample with schools as the first-stage sampling unit and students within schools as the second-stage unit. An average of 24 students in more than 1,000 public and private schools containing 8th grade students were sampled, yielding a sample size of approximately 25,000 8th graders. To date this sample has been resurveyed twice, in 1990 and 1992, when many of these youth were in the 10th and 12th grades, respectively. The study design calls for two more follow-ups, in 1994 and 1996, with the possibility of one or two additional follow-ups at two-year intervals (Davis and Sonnenberg, 1993). Thus, the current plans for the study involve following the NELS:88 8th grade cohort from approximately age 13 to at least age 21, and perhaps age 25.

In each of the three waves of NELS:88, sample respondents completed a questionnaire and a cognitive test battery. The student questionnaire gathered information regarding family background, language use, school experiences, work experiences, and plans for the future. During the base year of the study, a parent or guardian of the sampled student was asked to complete a questionnaire, as were two of the sampled students' teachers (in predetermined subject areas), as well as a school administrator. The parent questionnaire emphasized family background information, including parental status measures and parental involvement in and knowledge about their child's schooling; the teacher questionnaire examined teachers' perceptions of the sampled student's academic performance and personal qualities, the curriculum content of the courses they taught, and their background and beliefs about their work environment.

In addition to the student questionnaire and cognitive test battery, the first follow-up also included a school questionnaire (as many students changed schools in moving from the 8th grade to the 10th grade) and a teacher questionnaire, as well as a special questionnaire for school dropouts. The second follow-up included each of these kinds of instruments, as well as a parent questionnaire.

Since recent developments in the analysis of school effects have documented the importance of a "critical mass" of students within schools for reliable estimation, the NELS:88 sampling design presented potential analytic problems. In the NLS-72 and HS&B studies, the number of sampled students within high schools was fairly large, since high schools were the first-stage sampling units. But in NELS:88, the first-stage sampling unit was schools containing an 8th grade, many of which were middle or junior high schools. Consequently, many of the students in the study not only changed schools between the 8th and 10th grades, but also more importantly were spread more thinly among a large number of high schools.

Thus, many of the high schools attended by NELS:88 sample members contain only a handful of respondents. Recognizing this problem, NCES agreed to sponsor a School Effects Supplement, adding additional students and teachers to 250 of the high schools in the study. Although there are no base-year data (e.g., cognitive test scores) on these additional students, they do provide additional information for estimating school effects on secondary school experiences and outcomes.

The National Education Longitudinal Study of 1998

NCES is currently beginning the planning of the National Education Longitudinal Study of 1998 (NELS:98). Although the study design has yet to be determined, including the starting grade for the cohort of youth to be followed over time, it is expected that NELS:98 will resemble NELS:88 in its design and substantive foci. As with NELS:88, and HS&B, the NELS:98 study will examine the process by which young people move through the schooling system and into adult work and family roles. The most likely sources of data will once again be students themselves, their parents and teachers, and school administrators.

The Beginning Postsecondary Longitudinal Study

As noted above, when students cross school boundaries they frequently are more dispersed, so that a sampling design involving sizeable clusters of students at one level of schooling almost invariably results in small clusters of students at a higher level of schooling. Nowhere is this clearer than with the transition from secondary school to postsecondary education. As a consequence, NCES has initiated the Beginning Postsecondary Longitudinal Study (BPS), a study of a large, nationally representative cohort of students beginning postsecondary education. The BPS sample is drawn from the National Postsecondary Student Aid Study (NPSAS), a triennial cross-sectional study of students enrolled in a range of postsecondary institutions, including less-than-2-year institutions, community and junior colleges, 4-year colleges, and universities located across the country. The sample includes undergraduate, graduate, and professional school students, some of whom are receiving federally funded financial aid and others of whom are not. The purpose of BPS is to examine students' progress, persistence, and attainment of postsecondary education and their transitions between postsecondary education and work. By relying on a beginning cohort of postsecondary students, BPS will capture the experience of "nontraditional" (e.g., older) students as well as those who enter postsecondary schooling immediately or shortly after completing high school.

The first BPS cohort consists of about 7,000 students who began postsecondary schooling for the first time in the 1989-90 academic year and responded to the NPSAS:90 survey, which also gathered background and financial data from the parents of over 6,000 of these students. These students were resurveyed in 1992 and are scheduled to be followed up every two years. The base-year and follow-up surveys address students' postsecondary schooling and employment experiences, including academic progress, field of study, persistence, and future plans; family formation; and financial aid and expenses associated with postsecondary schooling. In addition, BPS will gather postsecondary transcripts. NCES anticipates drawing new BPS cohorts from every other NPSAS cohort, i.e., on a 6-year cycle (Davis and Sonnenberg, 1993).

NCES planning documents indicate that BPS is intended to focus on issues of progress and persistence in undergraduate education. Among the policy questions that BPS is intended to address are: How does the progress and persistence of nontraditional students differ from that of recent high school graduates? How does part-time or discontinuous attendance affect progress and persistence in postsecondary education? What is the modal rate of academic progress, and what educational experiences are related to making average progress toward completion? What is the match between postsecondary goals and attainments? What is the nature of postsecondary students' access to graduate and professional programs?

Although the planning documents are not clear on how long each BPS cohort will be followed, I suspect that the follow-ups are intended primarily to trace students' progress through postsecondary schooling and not much beyond that. Thus, the BPS study is not likely to be an important resource for understanding the labor force careers of current enrollees in postsecondary schooling. However, because sample members will be followed even if they leave postsecondary schooling early in the life of the study, BPS may be especially useful in monitoring the early labor market experiences of those postsecondary students who enter the labor force upon completion of 2-year postsecondary programs or other programs of limited duration.

The Baccalaureate and Beyond Longitudinal Study

Paralleling the BPS effort is another new NCES survey tied to NPSAS, called the Baccalaureate and Beyond Longitudinal Study (B&B). The first B&B cohort consists of 16,000 students completing their baccalaureate degrees in the 1992-93 academic year, a subsample of students surveyed in the cross-sectional 1993 NPSAS survey. The B&B study will resurvey this cohort at 1, 3, 6, 9, and 12-year intervals. For baccalaureate degree completers who are graduating at age 22, the follow-up period will span ages 23-34. Of course, some of the baccalaureate recipients in the B&B cohort will be older.

Because B&B will trace students' educational and occupational attainments for 12 years past the receipt of the baccalaureate degree, the study will contribute to our knowledge about postbaccalaureate schooling, including professional education, and the early labor force experience of highly educated youth, including estimates of the economic returns to advanced schooling. Since relatively few of the young people sampled in the other NCES longitudinal studies ever attend postbaccalaureate schooling, B&B will provide new information about the dynamics of progress and persistence in graduate and professional education.

As with BPS, the B&B study will rely on base-year NPSAS student and parent surveys, institutionally generated student records, and follow-up surveys of students. The data gathered will describe students' family backgrounds, including the financing of undergraduate and graduate education, educational experiences in undergraduate and graduate school, employment experience and family formation, and future expectations.

National Longitudinal Survey of Youth (NLSY) and Children of the NLSY

An important limitation of the studies noted above is their inability to link data on change and continuity in the family status of youth with their educational and occupational careers. Such studies typically provide little or no information on household composition or economic status prior to the base year of the survey, at which time respondents were in their early or late teens. They cannot therefore inform questions about the influence of persistent poverty or marital disruption on the educational attainment of youth.

A study that holds the promise of such analyses is the National Longitudinal Survey of Youth (NLSY). The NLSY is the fifth in a series of National Longitudinal Surveys of Labor Market Experience, currently administered by the Department of Labor's Bureau of Labor Statistics. As with its predecessors, it is a longitudinal study of the labor market experiences of a nationally representative cohort of individuals, in this case more than 12,000 noninstitutionalized civilian and military youth ages 14 to 21 in 1979. The survey oversampled black, Hispanic, and low-income white youth and has had extremely high response rates in the base year and subsequent follow-ups. The sample has been reinterviewed annually since the base year, although the military sample was discontinued in 1985 (Manser et al., 1990). To date, then, the NLSY cohort has been followed from age 14-21 to age 28-35.

As befitting a survey sponsored by the Bureau of Labor Statistics, the focus of the NLSY interviews is the employment experiences of respondents, including their sources of income, training, employment and unemployment spells, occupational mobility, and attitudes about and knowledge of work. Data are gathered on the dates of key events, a strategy that enables analysts to examine event histories. In addition, the interviews routinely ask about education and family formation and occasionally have included questions about child care, substance abuse, personal values, and career plans. The NLSY interviews have been supplemented by the High School Transcript Survey, sponsored by the National Center for Research in Vocational Education, and the Profiles of American Youth, sponsored by the Department of Defense, which administered the Armed Services Vocational Aptitude Battery to 94 percent of the sample (Manser et al., 1990).

Perhaps the most remarkable feature of the NLSY is the recent expansion of the study to include the children of the NLSY. In 1986, nearly 5,000 children of the civilian women in the NLSY sample were assessed, and most of these were reassessed in 1988 and 1990 (Chase-Lansdale et al., 1991). Although these children are not a nationally representative sample, since their mothers were on average younger when they were born than mothers in general, as the cohort of mothers ages and more children are added to the sample with succeeding births, the sample of children will eventually be representative of all children born to women ages 14-21 in 1979.

The sample size of older children remains rather small, but data reported in Chase-Lansdale et al. (1991) indicate that it now includes 300 youth age 17 or older, and in succeeding years this number will expand dramatically. Most of these youth will have completed a supplemental questionnaire intended to tap aspects of adolescent development, and younger children in the sample have already been assessed for their cognitive and socioemotional development with subscales of familiar psychological instruments.

Panel Study of Income Dynamics

The Panel Study of Income Dynamics (PSID) is a longitudinal study of families begun in 1968. The study has followed both the original families interviewed in 1968 and "split-off" families formed by individuals in those original families who subsequently left home and formed new families. These latter families include families formed when marriages dissolve and one or both partners form new households, and families formed when children leave home. Because the sample adds new families formed by children leaving home and discards families when all family members die, the resulting sample of families is unbiased (Duncan and Morgan, 1985).

The PSID has conducted annual interviews with the head of the household of all of the families in the sample, which in 1985 consisted of 6,500 families and 16,000 individuals (Duncan and Morgan, 1985). As might be surmised from the study's title, much of the data gathered pertain to sources of income in the calendar year preceding each interview, as well as detailed employment histories for the head of the household and partner and less-detailed data on the employment and earnings of other family members. The core data also include information on family composition, household expenditures, and housing (Duncan and Morgan, 1985). Other data have been gathered on a one-time or intermittent basis. Topics that have been covered at least once in the PSID interviews include child care information, disability and illness, job search strategies, unemployment, retirement plans and experience, savings patterns, and standardized test performance.

Because the core data are gathered annually, it is possible to form event histories for families and link them to the experiences of family members. The chapters in Elder (1985) provide examples of creative analytic efforts to model the consequences of variations in family experience (e.g., poverty status, marital stability, disability status) for families and their members. Of particular interest is the capacity to examine the effects of family background on children in longitudinal perspective.

There are, however, limits to the ways in which the PSID can inform our understanding of educational attainment and the transition into the labor force. Relatively few sample members are undergoing the transition to adulthood in a particular year, so that cross-sectional comparisons of the educational and occupational experiences of youth are not highly reliable. In addition, the data on family members who are not heads of households or their spouses are rather sketchy, so that data on adult children living at home are much thinner than data on similar youth who have formed independent households. Moreover, the data on children are reported by the household head rather than the children themselves, and thus are subject to some potential distortion.

SUMMARY STRENGTHS AND WEAKNESSES OF THE AVAILABLE DATA

Perhaps the most important point that one can make regarding the available sources of data on educational attainment and the transition into the labor force is that it is hard to characterize these data sources as a *system*. The data collections are administered by different agencies, each with its own substantive foci, and little thought has been given to how these differing data collections fit together or where the key redundancies and gaps might lie. No single organization has had the authority or the responsibility to manage the collection of information on educational attainment and the transition into the labor force. Consequently, the comparability of data gathered by different agencies, or even different branches *within* an agency, has been largely a hit-or-miss proposition. To be sure, communication has improved both across and within agencies, so that, for example, item wording is much less variable across surveys than it once was.

Nevertheless, it is clear that the existing data collection mechanisms fail to inform many important policy concerns about educational attainment and the transition into the labor force. I believe there are three major sources of slippage between the data that are gathered by the federal system and the data that might be most useful to policy makers: what questions are asked, when they are asked, and of whom they are asked.

What questions are asked? The foregoing discussion has suggested that a number of aspects of educational attainment and the transition to work are not well represented in the ongoing data collection system. Although the failure to ask the right questions may be seen as the source of the problem, it is important to understand that there are two very different reasons for the failure to ask the right questions. The first reason is what social scientists sometimes refer to specification error in models of social processes: the failure to include measures of theoretically relevant constructs in attempts to model or understand complex social phenomena.

Perhaps the most important model specification error in the studies reviewed above occurs when students' cognitive ability or knowledge is not taken into account. Because student learning is frequently correlated with students' schooling experiences and also is related to educational outcomes, the failure to take measured cognitive performance into account can lead to upwardly biased estimates of the effects of schooling experiences on such outcomes such as educational attainment. For example, the fact that youth who have been retained in grade in their primary or secondary school careers are more likely to drop out of school than those who have not does not necessarily imply that grade retention "causes" dropping out. Rather, it may simply be that those students who are struggling academically early in their schooling careers are both more likely to be held back and more likely to leave school before completion. It would, however, be extremely difficult to distinguish between these two possibilities without early data on students' cognitive performance.

The second kind of failure to ask the right questions stems from what social scientists refer to as measurement error. In this case, the relevant theoretical constructs are in fact represented in the data that are collected, but they are simply measured poorly. There is an ample number of examples of poorly measured variables in the datasets described earlier. Educational attainment, including when students were enrolled in school, and the kind of schooling in which they were enrolled, is measured unevenly in the studies I have reviewed, as is the quality of youth work experience. Even contextual factors such as family income or household configuration are subject to this criticism.

When are the questions asked? It is axiomatic that the periodicity of data collection needs to be calibrated with a theory of the stability or volatility of the phenomenon of interest. Phenomena that are known or presumed to be stable do not need to be measured frequently, whereas phenomena that change quickly over fairly short periods of time may need to be monitored repeatedly over that burst of time. We measure the unemployment rate monthly, because we know that those forces in the economy that affect employment and unemployment can change very rapidly, and in fact we *do* observe month-to-month variation in the unemployment rate that may exceed sampling variability. Conversely, a decennial youth unemployment measure would be of little use because it would likely miss most of the action from month to month and year to year. Yet it may not be meaningful to estimate a monthly dropout rate, because the forces that govern the dropout rate are not believed to shift from month to month. Annual or biennial data might be more appropriate, as a year or two is often the length of time before a new program or policy initiative starts to affect students in the way in which it was intended.

While I am not inclined to argue that any of the datasets reviewed earlier gather data too frequently, I do believe that there are instances in which the data collections are not frequent enough to allow for the meaningful monitoring of trends in educational attainment and the transition to work. In a context of relatively rapid educational reform and economic change, it may be desirable to address questions about high school completion, postsecondary access and persistence, and youth labor market experience as frequently as every two to three years. Those analytic questions depending on longitudinal data have typically relied on data from the NCES longitudinal studies, which have been spaced 8 to 10 years apart. This may simply be too long a time span to monitor changes in educational attainment and the transition to work.

To cite but one instance of this problem, one of the objectives associated with the Goal 2 of the National Education Goals pertains to the proportion of school dropouts who will return to complete a high school degree or its equivalent. Each of the three National Education Goals Reports—those issued in 1991, 1992, and 1993—has reported data on the percentage of High School and Beyond sophomores in 1980 who dropped out but then returned and completed high school by 1986. These data were already old when they were initially reported, but comparable data from the NELS:88 study, the subsequent NCES longitudinal study, will not be available until 1996.

Whereas the NCES longitudinal studies are exceedingly valuable, perhaps they need to be supplemented by more frequent short-term longitudinal studies focused on specific policy concerns, such as postsecondary access or the transition from high school to work. It may be advisable to assess trends in postsecondary access or persistence and their dependence on social background factors on a two- to three-year cycle. Such a hybrid strategy would retain the strengths of the NCES longitudinal studies program—especially the extraordinary diversity in the range of data gathered—while still providing more timely information on a smaller range of policy issues. Since these "gap" studies could not reflect the complexity of studies like HS&B and NELS:88, careful thought would have to be given to just what information is essential to gather to inform the most pressing policy concerns on a two- to three-year cycle.

Of whom are the questions asked? Implicit in the purpose of a workshop entitled "Integrating Federal Statistics on Children" is the presumption that such statistics can or should be integrated. Many of the important sources of data on children's well-being are sample surveys of households and their members who are followed through time. Of the data sources I have reviewed, only the NCES longitudinal studies are sensitive to the organizational context of schooling and work. If, as I have argued, organizational and institutional contexts are important in understanding educational attainment and the transition to work, then survey designs that are indifferent to these contexts may result in asking questions of the wrong people.

For example, questions about the effects of schools and their policies and programs on educational and labor market outcomes may require a sufficient number of students within schools to estimate those effects reliably. Household surveys typically are not designed to ensure a critical mass or cluster of individuals within a particular organizational context, such as a school or a firm. Even the NCES longitudinal studies, which by design sample students within schools, run into difficulties on this account, as students disperse when crossing grade levels or move from one school building to the next. It may be that we will need to depend on a synthetic cohort approach drawing on different cohorts at different levels of the education system (for example, NELS:88 coupled with BPS or B&B) to understand organizational and institutional influences on the educational and work careers of youth.

The important point here is, I believe, that the policy questions of interest should dictate study designs. Not all questions will be best addressed by household surveys, and some may warrant relatively unconventional sampling plans. We might imagine, for example, sampling youth working in specific firms that hire young people (e.g., fast food restaurants) or working in different sectors of the economy, thereby building important contextual comparisons into the study design.

There is an additional concern about who gets asked questions. Many of the important policy questions in the areas of educational attainment and youth employment pertain to the effectiveness of specific policies and programs. For example, we want to know what works in dropout prevention programs, or whether Upward Bound is successful in helping disadvantaged youth make the transition to postsecondary education. To what extent can the federal data system inform these questions?

The answer is, only a little. The broad federal statistical data collections that function as indicator systems are not a substitute for program evaluation. Evaluations of specific programs and policies typically require data that are tailored to understanding those programs and policies. Routine data collections are unlikely to ask the right questions of the right respondents. Targeted studies of particular programs and policies are a much more fruitful source of information about how such programs and policies work.

For example, the NELS:88 study asked school administrators to describe the dropout prevention programs in their schools and asked students both in and out of school about their experiences with such programs. But the questions are necessarily broad and vague and unlikely to delve sufficiently deeply into the characteristics of specific programs or into students' experiences with them to have much policy relevance. We can learn little about how programs are implemented, who they serve, and how effective they are from the broad social surveys that make up the current federal data system.

Conversely, there are other mechanisms for gathering information that might address such policy concerns. For example, the Office of Planning and Policy in the U.S. Department of Education is sponsoring an evaluation of the School Dropout Demonstration Assistance Program, a federally funded demonstration program involving 65 sites around the country, conducted by Mathematica Policy Research. The data gathered through this evaluation will not be linked to any of the data sources I have described, but they will bear directly on issues in the implementation and impact of model dropout prevention programs.

COVERAGE OF SUBPOPULATIONS OF POLICY RELEVANCE

In light of historic concerns about equality of opportunity, both educational and otherwise, the datasets described previously are often used to examine the status of traditionally disadvantaged populations—racial/ethnic minorities, the poor, women, and, more recently, language minority and disabled children and youth. Although the issue of the adequacy of the coverage of such subpopulations in these datasets is necessarily subjective, there are two general points to be made.

First, some studies exclude policy-relevant subpopulations by design. The CPS, for example, excludes institutionalized youth, who are likely to be disproportionately poor and minority. Similarly, the NCES longitudinal studies have omitted early school-leavers by design, as the NLS-72 began with a cohort of high school seniors, and HS&B with cohorts of seniors and sophomores. These studies provided limited knowledge about school dropouts in general and early school dropouts in particular.

Second, given the designs and sample sizes of most of the data collections reviewed here, subpopulations that are relatively rare in the population are unlikely to be studied reliably without substantial oversampling. Minority racial or ethnic group members, language minority youth, and disabled youth represent relatively small shares of the youth population and thus may not be represented in study samples in sufficient numbers to estimate their experiences reliably. Some studies have oversampled several small groups of policy interest. For example, the NELS:88 study oversampled Hispanic and Asian and Pacific Islander students, as well as mainstreamed hearing-impaired students enrolled in Individualized Education Programs. Often, though, such sample augmentations are dependent on an outside agency providing supplemental funds. In the case of NELS:88, the Hispanic and Asian and Pacific Islander sample augmentation was funded by the Office of Bilingual Education and Minority Language Affairs in the Department of Education, and the sample of hearing-impaired students by Gallaudet University.

STRATEGIES FOR IMPROVING THE CAPACITY OF THE FEDERAL STATISTICAL SYSTEM TO ADDRESS INFORMATION NEEDS

I conclude this brief review by asking how we might increase the capacity of the federal statistical system to address the needs of policy makers for data on the well-being of children and youth. This is no mean task, given the historic fragmentation and politicization of the federal statistical system. I have no sure-fire strategies to suggest—simply some provisional suggestions.

1. Conduct a needs assessment. A necessary first step is to understand the information needs of policy makers, the terrain of the available data, and the quality of the fit between the two. The workshop for which this paper has been prepared is an excellent first step in mapping out what is known and what is needed, and the selection of agency professionals, contractors, and academics as discussants broadens the base of the discussion. I believe the discourse over what is needed and what is available should be broadened even further to include agency executives in key policy-making roles (e.g., the assistant secretary for postsecondary education), legislative committee members and/or their staffs, the major advocacy groups (e.g., the Children's Defense Fund), professional associations (e.g., the American Educational Research Association), and the think tanks that represent a key

consumer group for federal data relevant to policy (e.g., the Urban Institute).

2. Convene an interagency working group composed of the agencies responsible for the production, dissemination and analysis of federal statistics bearing on the well-being of children and youth to examine gaps, overlaps, and redundancies in the federal statistical system. Such a working group could take the proceedings of this workshop as a point of departure. In my view, it would be essential for the working group to have the necessary technical expertise to examine the plausible budgetary implications of alternatives to existing data collections. It also would be crucial to have the Office of Management and Budget represented in this working group, in light of its oversight role for the collection of federal data.

3. Lodge oversight responsibility for the federal data system as it bears on the well-being of children and youth in an individual or group that has the capacity to hold the agencies' feet to the fire and arbitrate among different agency interests. As I have noted earlier in this paper, the distinctive histories and constituencies of the various federal agencies that gather statistics on children and youth must be taken into account in trying to understand why the system looks the way it does. Agencies occasionally are in competition for the responsibility to gather certain kinds of data, and perenially they are in competition, whether direct or indirect, for the scarce federal dollars devoted to statistics. There seems to be a need for an oversight body that can rise above the individual and sometimes competing interests of particular agencies and shape a federal data system that is responsive to the full spectrum of policy concerns about children and youth, particularly those concerns that cross traditional agency boundaries.

These are some possible action steps, but I am uneasy about concluding this paper without questioning one of the fundamental assumptions that undergirds it and the workshop for which it was prepared. I believe that the federal statistics system can be a useful tool for policy makers concerned with educational attainment and the transition to work in particular, and the well-being of children and youth in general. But statistics, and the surveys and censuses that generate them, are just one part of a portfolio of data sources that can be useful. It is important to keep in mind that there are many important policy issues concerning the well-being of children and youth that are better addressed through delimited program evaluations, qualitative case studies, and other modes of social science analysis that do not produce statistical estimates with known precision. In the absence of powerful theories of how the education system and the labor market work, we need to draw on as many defensible sources of knowledge as we can. It would be a shame if attention to the statistics system were to diminish the interest in other sources of social science evidence regarding how children and youth negotiate the transition to adulthood.

REFERENCES

Alexander, K.L., A.M. Pallas, and S. Holupka
1987 Consistency and change in educational stratification: recent trends regarding social background and college access. Pp. 161-185 in R. Robinson, ed., *Research in Social Stratification and Mobility, Volume 6.* Greenwich, Conn.: JAI Press.

Bureau of Labor Statistics
1988 *BLS Handbook of Methods, Bulletin 2285.* Washington, D.C.: U.S. Government Printing Office.

Charner, I., and B.S. Fraser
1988 *Youth and Work: What We Know, What We Don't Know, What We Need to Know.* Washington, D.C.: The William T. Grant Foundation on Work, Family and Citizenship.

Chase-Lansdale, P.L., F.L. Mott, J. Brooks-Gunn, and D.A. Phillips
1991 Children of the National Longitudinal Survey of Youth: a unique research opportunity. *Developmental Psychology* 27:918-931.

Chubb, J., and T. Moe
1990 *Politics, Markets, and America's Schools.* Washington, D.C.: The Brookings Institution.

Davis, C., and B. Sonnenberg, eds.
1993 *Programs and Plans of the National Center for Education Statistics, 1993 Edition.* Washington, D.C.: U.S. Government Printing Office.

Duncan, G., and J. Morgan
1985 The Panel Study of Income Dynamics. In G.H. Elder, Jr., ed., *LifeCourse Dynamics: Trajectories and Transitions, 1968-1980.* Ithaca, N.Y.: Cornell University Press.

Ekstrom, R.B., M.E. Goertz, and D.A. Rock
1988 *Education and American Youth.* London: Falmer Press.

Elder, G.H., Jr.
1985 *Life Course Dynamics: Trajectories and Transitions, 1968-1980.* Ithaca, N.Y.: Cornell University Press.

Hauser, R.M.
1991 Trends in College Entry Among Whites, Blacks, and Hispanics, 1972-1988. Discussion Paper No. 958-91. Institute for Research on Poverty, University of Wisconsin, Madison.

Kaufman, P., M. McMillen, and D. Bradby
1992 *Dropout Rates in the United States: 1991.* Washington, D.C.: National Center for Education Statistics.

Kominski, R., and P.M. Siegel
1993 Measuring education in the Current Population Survey. *Monthly Labor Review* September:34-38.

Kominski, Robert
1990 Estimating the national high school dropout rate. *Demography* 27:303-311.

Manser, M., M. Pergamit, and W.B. Peterson
1990 National longitudinal surveys: development and uses. *Monthly Labor Review* July:32-37.

Mizell, H.
1988 A commentary on Ivan Charner and Bryna Shore Fraser's Youth and Work: What We Know, What We Don't Know, What We Need to Know. Pp. 97-106 in I. Charner and B.S. Fraser, *Youth and Work: What We Know, What We Don't Know, What We Need to Know*. Washington, D.C.: The William T. Grant Foundation on Work, Family and Citizenship.

OERI Goal 2 Work Group
1994 *Reaching the Goals: Goal 2—High School Completion*. Washington, D.C.: Office of Educational Research and Improvement, U.S. Department of Education.

Polivka, A.E., and J.M. Rothgeb
1993 Redesigning the CPS questionnaire. *Monthly Labor Review* September:10-28.

Rosenbaum, J.E., T. Kariya, R. Settersten, and T. Maier
1990 Market and network theories of the transition from high school to work: their application to industrialized societies. *Annual Review of Sociology* 16:263-299.

Wilson, W.J.
1987 *The Truly Disadvantaged: The Inner City, The Underclass, and Public Policy*. Chicago: University of Chicago Press.

Monitoring Changes in Health Care for Children and Families

Paul Newacheck and Barbara Starfield

INTRODUCTION

In 1994, when the workshop on integrating federal statistics on children was held, health care reform was a leading item on the agendas of the Clinton administration and the Congress. Although federal legislative progress in this area is now uncertain, the concern of many stakeholders over access, costs, and quality of the health care system is driving change at the state level. Indeed, several states have already moved to implement health care reforms. In addition, powerful economic forces are leading to rapid changes in the organization and delivery of health care. For example, the move throughout the country to managed health care in the private sector is one indication of the kind of reform that may gather strength, with or without federal legislation. These changes and others in the health care system are the result of several factors.

Paul Newacheck is at the Institute for Health Policy Studies, University of California at San Francisco. Barbara Starfield is at the Department of Health Policy and Management, Johns Hopkins University.

This paper was drafted and presented in 1994, when proposals for health care reform were being put forward and debated by the Clinton administration and in Congress. The authors have revised the text somewhat to reflect changing circumstances. However, the implications for federal statistics on children of eventual changes in the nation's health care system remain significant.

First, the high and rapidly growing costs of the health care system have generated concerns about the tax burdens of public programs such as Medicaid and Medicare, threats to the competitiveness of industry as a result of the high costs of employee health benefits, high administrative costs associated with a disorganized mechanism of paying for services through uncoordinated insurance policies, and perverse incentives for the use of unnecessary technology.

Second, access to basic health care services remains problematic for millions of people as a result of poorly distributed personnel and facilities, lack of insurance and inadequate insurance coverage for a substantial proportion of the population (especially children and young adults), cost sharing that imposes a barrier to seeking needed health services, employment insecurity and the lack of portability of insurance coverage with changes in place of employment, and the refusal of many health care providers to deliver services to individuals covered by public programs such as Medicaid.

Third, there is continuing concern about the availability, quality, and effectiveness of care as reflected by the relatively poor performance of the United States on major health indicators (especially among the young) and evidence of lack of effectiveness of many health services interventions.

Fourth, persistent and perhaps growing inequities among subgroups of the population have resulted from systematic differences in access to care and quality of care, insurance mechanisms such as experience rating, in which the sickest and most disadvantaged are less able to obtain insurance, and a premium structure for health insurance that requires the least well off to pay as much as the wealthiest for their health insurance coverage.

Health care reforms are likely to bring about profound changes in the manner in which children and their families in this country obtain health care. Universal coverage would give almost 10 million children who are now uninsured health insurance coverage (Snider and Boyce, 1994). Millions more would be likely to see improvements in the breadth and depth of their coverage. Others would see their coverage become more restrictive or their choice of providers become more limited.

Under managed competition, the approach favored by the president and many in Congress, there would be an acceleration of the already rapid growth of managed care arrangements, such as health maintenance organizations and preferred provider organizations. Managed care offers important potential for reducing costs and improving access to quality care. Yet many urge caution regarding the rapid adoption of managed care because of the financial incentives to underserve patients in prepaid systems of care (Newacheck et al., 1994; Fox and McManus, 1992).

Although little research has been conducted to date on the effects of managed care on children, it is clear that customary doctor-patient relationships will be disrupted for many families as they enter organized systems of care. Proponents of managed care argue that access to primary care will be facilitated; however, it is not clear that this would be the case. Access to specialist services would almost certainly be reduced in managed care settings. Pediatricians would increasingly be asked to serve as gatekeepers for the service system; at the same time they would experience reduced autonomy in choosing courses of treatment for their patients.

Beyond these direct effects on pediatric patients and providers, health care reforms carry significant indirect ramifications for families. For example, some families would see their out-of-pocket expenses for medical care decline, freeing resources for other family needs. Other families would experience increased outlays for medical care. Changes occurring under health care reform would also reverberate in the labor market. Most health care reform proposals would end the practice of imposing preexisting condition clauses in insurance policies. These restrictive clauses, common in health insurance plans offered through small employers, can circumscribe job mobility for families with disabled children. The effect of eliminating this practice would be profound, since 4 million American children now suffer from disabling chronic conditions (Benson and Marano, 1994).

It is less clear how the myriad special programs serving vulnerable populations of children would be affected by health care reform. The federal government now helps to fund a network of over 500 community and migrant health centers across the United States. Low-income families and their children often seek care in these and other publicly sponsored health centers and clinics. In addition, the federal government currently spends upward of $500 million annually on maternal and child health block grants. The states supplement these grants with their own funds to operate a variety of programs serving low-income and other children with special needs. Federal, state, and local governments also support emergency medical services for children, regionalized systems of prenatal care, regional centers serving children with rare chronic diseases, family planning programs, and other services. The fate of these programs and others that make up the public health system remains uncertain.

Monitoring and evaluating the changes that accompany health care reforms for children, their families, and the health care system that serves them presents a formidable challenge. Fortunately, the United States possesses a system for collecting and disseminating health statistics that is the envy of most other developed countries. Even so, our health statistics programs were not designed for the purpose of monitoring and evaluating health care reform. Consequently, an assessment of their utility for this purpose is in order.

In doing so, it is important to keep in mind that changes in the health care system will not affect all populations in the same manner. Children's health needs and provider networks differ from those of adults. Children's illnesses and injuries are diagnosed and treated in the context of rapid growth and developmental processes that have no counterpart in adults. Their physiological, cognitive, and emotional maturation makes children uniquely vulnerable to certain illnesses. Their developmental vulnerabilities require heightened attention to preventive care and early diagnosis and treatment of their disorders (Jameson and Wehr, 1993). Assessment of the current federal health statistics programs and the design of mechanisms for monitoring the effects of changes in the system must take into account these differences.

In the next section, a framework is presented for assessing the types of data needed for monitoring the effects of health care reforms on children and families.

DATA NEEDED FOR MONITORING CHANGES IN HEALTH CARE

Evaluation of the changing health care system requires data that systematically address concerns about equity, access, quality, and costs of care. Timely and reliable data are needed to support the administration and operations of the health care system, to measure the performance of providers, ensure quality, and support public health objectives and programs (Gaus et al., 1993).

Table 1 provides a framework for considering the data elements that are required, over time, and at the different levels at which health policies and planning are generated. The table also indicates the types of data sources required to obtain the needed information. Examples of the types of data needed for monitoring changes in health care for children, families, and the health care system are presented below in narrative form.

- Information is needed to ascertain the state of health and functional status of the population; the adequacy of access for preventive, curative, palliative, and rehabilitative services; barriers to the receipt of care; the equity of use of services across different population groups; and the degree to which services are distributed where they are most needed. Information concerning the burden of cost sharing and the degree to which it interferes with the receipt of needed services; the extent to which the goals of continuity and coordination of care are achieved; and satisfaction of the population with perceived technical, interpersonal, and organizational aspects of health service are also needed. The indirect costs of illness, such as time lost from work and school and child care costs attributable to illness, are also important.
- Information about the services provided is needed to ascertain the

TABLE 1 Data Elements Needed for Monitoring and Evaluating Health Care Reform

Units of Analysis	Domains	Indicators	Data Sources
Populations	Access to care	Insurance coverage (including covered and uncovered services), sources of primary care and specialty services, travel time, appointment waiting time, office waiting time, unmet needs, barriers to care	Population surveys
	Health care utilization	Hospitalizations; number and types of visits to different kinds of physicians and other health professionals; long-term care; use of medications, medical equipment, and supplies; perceived quality of services; continuity, coordination of, and comprehensiveness of services; satisfaction with services	Population surveys; provider surveys
	Health care expenditures	Total and out-of-pocket personal health care expenditures, including hospital, physicians, mental health, other professional services, long-term care, medications, medical equipment and supplies. Indirect costs of illness.	Population surveys; administrative records
	Health status	Infant and childhood mortality, low birthweight, health and functional status indicators (including physical, development, behavioral, and emotional), restricted activity days, indicators of risks, and resilience to illness	Vital statistics; population surveys; surveillance data

Health plans and providers	Health care services	Presenting problems, diagnosis, case mix; degree to which care is comprehensive, coordinated, and continuous; adequacy of prenatal infant, childhood, and adolescent care; provision of appropriate immunizations and other preventive services; frequency of well-child examinations, quality of care for individual acute and chronic conditions	Population surveys; provider surveys; administrative records
	Effectiveness of care	Reasons for visits, health services interventions (including procedures, tests, medications and other therapies (including home health care), referrals, organizational amenities (such as waiting times); types of practitioners involved in providing services; outcomes of visits	Population surveys; administrative records
Health systems	Health care resources	Work force deployment, by type of professional and type of physician; primary care resources; specialty care resources; hospitals; ambulatory care organizations (including HMOs); long-term care facilities, laboratories; home health services organizations, public health organizations & services, (e.g., school health facilities)	Systems surveillance
	Health care expenditures	System-level health care expenditures, mode of financing; mode of payments; expenditures by type of service	System surveillance

extent and type of health care needs being served; the distribution of services; the extent to which practice patterns are targeted to the needs of the population served; the extent to which they are organized to provide care that is accessible, comprehensive, continuous, and coordinated; and the extent to which the services provided are justified by evidence of effectiveness and appropriateness.

• Information about the organization and distribution of resources within the health care system is needed in order to plan and monitor their adequacy and equity with regard to preventive services, primary care services, and consultative and referral services. Of importance are the deployment of practitioners and facilities, the mode of financing and the distribution of payments for services, the availability of primary care (for both physical and mental child health problems) and specialty services for children with chronic health problems, and the availability and deployment of special modes of intervention such as home visiting, medications, and devices where they are needed. Information concerning the costs of care provided and the sources of payments for various aspects of care is required in order to discern the degree of success in maintaining cost control within the health services system. Information is also needed to determine the balance of expenditures between primary care and specialty care as well as between preventive care and care of illness.

• Information is also needed to track environmental and social characteristics that predispose children and families to illness or interfere with efforts to ameliorate illness.

Data collection strategies should be designed to provide baseline information on all of these characteristics and should be organized to monitor changes over time as health care reforms are implemented. Planning for information retrieval should be coordinated so that data collected at local levels can be aggregated to the regional, state, and federal level, and so that data collected at higher levels can be related to data collected at lower levels. This will permit comparisons to be made across health plans, geographic regions, and states and will enable health planners to identify more successful models for delivery of care from ones that are less successful in meeting the objectives of reform.

In the next section, the major existing sources of data are identified and evaluated against the information needs (outlined above) for evaluating changes in health care.

CHARACTERISTICS OF CURRENT DATA SOURCES

There are approximately 500 health, social, and demographic data projects in the U.S. Department of Health and Human Services alone. Added to these are state and local data collection efforts, projects of private groups, and administrative and clinical databases of health facilities, plans, and insurance agencies. Evaluation of health care reforms will require a change in thinking about the locus of control for health data systems. Since both governmental and private data sources are needed to address the variety of characteristics in Table 1, a public-private partnership in developing the framework and mechanisms for data collection and analysis is a critical goal.

In this section, the major federal, state, and private data collection efforts are presented and discussed with regard to their current contributions to knowledge as well as changes that are required in order to make them more suitable for evaluation of health care reforms.

Table 1 listed the types of data sources for obtaining information from populations, providers and health care plans, and health systems. Table 2 provides brief descriptions of major databases relevant to monitoring changes in health care. And it is organized according to these types of information sources:

- Vital statistics and surveillance systems for obtaining population-based information concerning health status.
- Population surveys to obtain data concerning health status, access to services, use of services, experiences and satisfaction with various aspects of services, and both direct and indirect out-of-pocket costs of dealing with health problems.
- Provider surveys to obtain information on the characteristics of services used, types of services provided, distribution of facilities, and types of health conditions diagnosed.
- Administrative records from health plans and providers for providing information on the adequacy of arrangements for assessing health care needs of populations served, characteristics of care provided (including the balance between primary care and specialty care, as well as between preventive, curative, palliative, and rehabilitative aspects of care), the resources expended in providing care, the adequacy of organizational arrangements for achieving comprehensive, continuous, and coordinated care, documentation of effectiveness of care provided, and costs generated in the provision of services.
- Health systems data to determine the distribution of facilities and personnel and their type, the sources of funding for the provision of services, the distribution of expenditures by type and source of care, and total expenditures for providing care to population groups differing in the extent and type of their health care needs.

An additional category of data addresses documentation of environmen-

TABLE 2 Population-Based Data Sources for Monitoring Children's Health Status

Name and Sponsor	Data Source/ Methods	Selected Applications of Data for Health Care Reform
A. Vital Statistics and Surveillance		
Vital Statistics Cooperative Program (NCHS)	State vital registration	Life expectancy; causes of death; infant mortality; prenatal care and birthweight; birth rates; teenage and unmarried births; family formation and dissolution; pregnancy outcomes
Linked Birth/ Infant Death Program (NCHS)	Birth and death certificates	Infant mortality rates by birth cohort; infant mortality rates by birthweight
National Death Index (NCHS)	Death certificates	Facilitates epidemiologic follow-up studies; verification of death for individuals under study; most NCHS surveys are linked to NDI
Youth Risk Behavior Surveillance System (CDC)	Self-administered questionnaire in schools	Assessment of changes in health practices over time
B. Population Surveys		
National Health Interview Survey (NCHS)	Personal interviews	Large-scale data set with ability to establish trends in access, utilization, and health status
National Health Interview Survey on Child and Family Health (NCHS)	Personal interviews	Health status; chronic conditions; behavioral problems; learning and developmental problems; birth characteristics

Overall Sample	Child/Family Sample	Planned Periodicity
All births, deaths, and fetal deaths; sample of marriages and divorces; termination of pregnancy for selected reporting areas	All births, deaths, and fetal deaths; sample of marriages and divorces; termination of pregnancy for selected reporting areas	Annual
All U.S. births and infant deaths	All U.S. births and infant deaths	Annual
All deaths	All deaths occurring among children	Annual
Nationally representative sample of students in grades 9-12; state-level data available	Only adolescents surveyed; comparable but unlinked survey data for adults	Every 2 years
50,000 households	Approximately 30,000 children under 18 years plus family members	Annual; insurance and access surveys added in 1993
One child from each NHIS household	17,000 children (in 1988) under 18 years plus linked data on other family members	Every 7-8 years; planned for 1996 if funding available

continued on next page

TABLE 2 Continued

Name and Sponsor	Data Source/ Methods	Selected Applications of Data for Health Care Reform
National Maternal Infant Health Survey (NCHS)	Follow-back using state vital records; interviews of mothers; hospital medical records; prenatal care providers	Factors associated with low birthweight and infant death; barriers to prenatal care; effects of maternal risk factors on pregnancy outcomes
National Survey of Family Growth (NCHS)	Personal interviews; telephone interviews	Contraception and sterilization; teenage sexual activity and pregnancy; family planning and unintended pregnancy; adoption; infertility
National Health and Nutrition Examination Survey	Personal interviews; physical examinations; laboratory tests	Physical health; clinical findings; growth and development
National Medical Expenditure Survey (AHCPR)	Multiple personal interviews; provider record checks; insurance policies analysis	Linked data on access, utilization, health status, and expenditures
National Longitudinal Survey of Youth-Child Data (DOL and NICHD)	Personal interviews	Longitudinal tracking of health status
Early Childhood Longitudinal Survey (NCES)	Personal interviews with parents and children; school questionnaire; teacher questionnaire	Longitudinal tracking of access, utilization, and health status

Overall Sample	Child/Family Sample	Planned Periodicity
10,000 live births; 4,000 fetal deaths; 6,000 infant deaths; oversample of blacks	10,000 live births; 4,000 fetal deaths; 6,000 infant deaths	Every 8 years, with longitudinal follow-up; last conducted in 1988 with 1991 follow-up
8,500 women ages 15-44; oversample of blacks	8,500 women ages 15-44; oversample of blacks	Every 5 years subsequent follow-up; last conducted in 1988 with 1990 telephone interviews
30,000 persons ages 2 months and older examined for NHANES III	14,000 children under age 20	Periodic; currently in 4th year of 6-year cycle; continuous examinations to begin in 1996
14,000 households	10,500 children (in 1987) plus linked data on other family members	Every 8-10 years; last conducted in 1987; planned for 1996
Children born to female members of the NLSY	Approximately 8,500 children	Every 2 years
A cohort of 23,000 kindergarten children	A cohort of 23,000 kindergarten children	Will follow cohort through 5th grade; data collection to begin with 1998-1999 school year

continued on next page

TABLE 2 Continued

Name and Sponsor	Data Source/ Methods	Selected Applications of Data for Health Care Reform
Survey of Income and Program Participation (Census)	Personal interviews	Longitudinal tracking of program participation, health insurance coverage, and health status
Survey of Program Dynamics (Census)	Personal interviews	Longitudinal tracking of access, utilization, and health status
Current Population Survey (Census)	Personal interviews	Health insurance coverage; public program participation
National Household Survey on Drug Abuse (ADAMHA)	Sample survey of population age 12 and older	Prevalence of substance abuse
C. Provider Surveys		
National Hospital Discharge Surveys (NCHS)	Hospital records; computerized data sources	Patient characteristics; length of stay; diagnosis and multiple diagnoses; surgical and diagnostic procedures
National Survey of Ambulatory Surgery (NCHS)	Abstract forms completed by facility staff	Patient characteristics; diagnosis and multiple diagnoses; surgical and diagnostic procedures
National Ambulatory Medical Care Survey (NCHS)	Encounter forms completed by physicians practicing in private offices	Characteristics of patients' visits to physicians; diagnoses and treatment

Overall Sample	Child/Family Sample	Planned Periodicity
32-month longitudinal panel survey; 20,000 households	15,000 children under age 18 in 1990 panel	A new panel is introduced every 12 months; beginning 1996, a 48-month panel of 50,000 households is planned
20,000 households from the 1993 SIPP panel	Approximately 15,000 children	Will follow over a 10-year period if funding available
57,000 households monthly	33,000 children under age 15	Monthly; health insurance and program participation data collected in March surveys
18,000 households	Approximately 5,000 youth ages 12-17	Biennial
494 hospitals; 274,000 discharges	Approximately 60,000 discharge records for children under 18 years	Annual
700 facilities; 180,000 patient records	Unknown (to be implemented in 1994)	Annual; to be implemented in 1994
3,400 physicians in office-based practices; 45,000 patient visits	Approximately 7,500 records for children	Annual

continued on next page

TABLE 2 Continued

Name and Sponsor	Data Source/ Methods	Selected Applications of Data for Health Care Reform
National Home and Hospice Care Survey (NCHS)	Questionnaires completed by home health agencies and hospices	Number of patients; functional status of patients; number of discharged patients; characteristics of home health agencies and hospices and their patients
National Hospital Ambulatory Medical Care Survey (NCHS)	Encounter forms completed by physicians and other hospital staff	Characteristics of patients' visits in hospital outpatient departments and emergency departments; diagnoses and treatment
National Employer Health Insurance Survey (NCHS)	Computer-assisted telephone interviewing	State-level estimates of private health insurance; detailed national-level analysis of private health insurance; characteristics of employer spending for health care
Healthcare Cost and Utilization Project (AHCPR)	State hospital discharge records from public and private systems	Hospital utilization; variation in practice patterns
D. Administrative Records		
National Health Provider Inventory (NCHS)	Health care facilities; state licensing agencies; professional associations	Characteristics of hospitals, nursing and related care homes, hospices, and home health agencies; sampling frame for provider surveys
Claims Data	Claims submitted to private insurance companies for insured individuals and claims submitted to state Medicaid agencies	Hospitalization; quality of care; variation in practice patterns; health care payments; diagnosis and treatments; some data have cost sharing

Overall Sample	Child/Family Sample	Planned Periodicity
1,500 home health agencies and hospices; 7,000 current patients; 7,000 discharged patients	Approximately 700 records for children under 18 years	Annual
525 hospitals; 70,000 patient visits	Approximately 15,000 records for children under age 15	Annual
Stratified national sample of establishments to include all sizes of businesses, both private and public sector; 100,000 establishments screened to conduct 51,000 interviews	Not applicable	Annual; to be implemented in 1994
Hospital discharge records from 14 state data systems	Depends on state	Continuous data collection effort funded through 1994
All licensed/certified facilities in covered categories	Not applicable	Periodic; recently expanded to include additional providers
Depends on system	Depends on system	Depends on system

continued on next page

TABLE 2 Continued

Name and Sponsor	Data Source/ Methods	Selected Applications of Data for Health Care Reform
State Hospital Discharge Data	Approximately 20 states	Resources expended; medical practice; variations
Tape to Tape Medicaid Files (HCFA)	Medicaid enrollment, claims, and provider-level data from selected states	Hospitalization and ambulatory care visits; quality of care; variation in practice patterns
E. System Surveillance		
Area Resource File	Compilation of other data sources	Health personnel, health facilities, utilization data; relationships between services provided and area resources available

ADAMHA Alcohol, Drug, and Mental Health Administration
AHCPR Agency for Health Care Policy and Research
Census Bureau of the Census
CDC Centers for Disease Control and Prevention
DOL Department of Labor

tal and social characteristics that have an impact on health and responsiveness to medical interventions. These data sources are generally maintained by public health and human services agencies at the federal, state, regional, and local levels. Since the relevance and usefulness of these data sources extend beyond personal health services, they are not separately reviewed in this section.

Below, we describe the principal sources of data for monitoring changes in health care.

Vital Statistics and Surveillance Data

Vital statistics provide the means to describe changes in the rates and causes of death and some major causes of morbidity in the population. Many but not all sources of vital statistics contain information that enable

Overall Sample	Child/Family Sample	Planned Periodicity
All hospitals in selected states	Data on hospitalizations only; individuals not traceable	Continuous
Enrollment and claims forms and provider data from 5 states	Enrollees in 5 states	Continuous
Data derived from multiple surveys and administrative data systems	Same data specifically relevant for children, e.g., births to teenagers; no individual-level data	Continually updated

HCFA Health Care Financing Administration
NICHD National Institute for Child Health and Human Development
NCES National Center for Education Statistics
NCHS National Center for Health Statistics

analysts to detect differences (primarily concerning race and selected socioeconomic characteristics) among major population subgroups in order to identify possible sources of inequity in the provision of services. Greater specificity in relating differences in rates of preventable mortality and morbidity to differences in the use of medical services depends on linking these vital statistics to other sources of information. In some cases, these other sources of information are vital statistics themselves. For example, linked birth-death records provide a means to examine the relationship between infant mortality (from death certificates) and prenatal care (often contained on birth records). In other instances, linkages must be made with other types of data. For example, when linked with the Area Resource File (a system surveillance dataset), vital statistics can provide information on the relationship between preventable mortality or morbidity and the level of resources available in the same geographic area. It should be noted, however, that relationships that are uncovered by these types of analyses are "structure-outcome" or ecological relationships. That is, they provide only circumstantial evidence of a relationship, since information to assess the "process" by which the availability of resources influences the outcome is unavailable (Starfield, 1973). As noted below, one of the most marked deficits in existing information systems is the general absence of linkages that make it possible to determine the specific impact of different types of health resources on health.

The major contribution of vital statistics to date has been to facilitate epidemiologic studies of the influence of some important sociodemographic characteristics on mortality and morbidity and the elucidation of time trends that are ecologically associated with the availability of system resources. With the establishment of a means of linking most surveys sponsored by the National Center for Health Statistics to the death certificates through the National Death Index, it is now possible to explore the relationship between an even wider variety of individual characteristics and death from different causes.

Since most vital statistics are available in comparable form in other industrialized nations, international comparisons carried out at specific times or across time have been useful in identifying possible relationships between major health system characteristics and vital events. If linkages between vital statistics and sources of information on practice characteristics were developed, it would be possible for the first time to evaluate the direct impact of health services on major aspects of health.

Surveillance data, such as immunization surveys, case registries, the Pregnancy Risk Assessment Monitoring System, the Behavioral Risk Factor Surveillance Study, and the Youth Risk Behavior Surveillance System, are generally most useful when certain types of problems arise and are of great concern. They are helpful in pointing to directions for changes in public policy, including the need for new funding and more targeted delivery of specific services. Since they are limited to information on the specific issue of concern, they have limited long-term applicability to overall health system reform. As the development of data systems for health care reforms progresses, it might be possible to adopt data elements from these surveillance activities for routine incorporation into ongoing surveys, reserving the full surveillance surveys for detection of long-term trends by administration every few years.

Population Surveys

Almost all national population-based health surveys focus heavily on health status and utilization of health services. Household surveys commonly obtain information on number of hospitalizations and physician visits, and some collect information on use of other professional services. Most also obtain information on self-reported health status, and at least one survey provides physical examination data. Some also address insurance coverage and enrollment in or receipt of services from special programs that are government-administered or administered privately. Less frequently, household surveys are fielded to collect information on total and out-of-pocket expenses for health services.

Despite the apparent duplication of information obtained by different agencies in their survey efforts, few surveys attempt to obtain information concerning the types of health services that are sought (especially with regard to the distinction between primary and consultative services), the reasons for individual visits to physicians and other health personnel, the characteristics of those visits as reported by individuals, and the perceived outcomes of those visits. Most surveys are cross-sectional, making it impossible to track health status or experiences with the health system over time to determine changes that might be related to use of services. Furthermore, the validity of specific questions concerning health status is largely untested. When the National Health Interview Survey was first initiated, major efforts were made to determine the validity of information about reported doctor visits and hospitalizations. For the most part, however, questions concerning reported chronic conditions among children are of unknown accuracy, as are questions on acute disability and limitations of activity. Although a major methodological study comparing household survey data and medical record data on chronic conditions was recently conducted for adults, children were excluded from the study (Edwards et al., 1994). Until methodological studies begin to include children, survey results will remain of unknown accuracy.

Health surveys in the era of health care reform must be able to discern the impact of health services on perceived and documented health status. Health status, as determined from surveys, is composed of many different characteristics reflecting diagnosed conditions ("condition lists"), acute disability (as determined by restrictions on usual activities due to acute or chronic conditions), and long-term limitations of activity due to chronic conditions. Only infrequently is the presence of symptoms ascertained. Mental health symptoms, in the rare instances in which they are elicited, are generally treated as separate and distinct from physical symptoms and conditions, despite the recognition among mental health professionals that they are interrelated (Leginski et al., 1989). Indeed, even when data on mental and physical health are collected in the same survey, it can be impossible to assess joint occurrence. This was the case with the 1988 National Health Interview Survey on Child Health. Useful questions were asked about physical, emotional, developmental, and learning problems, but different reference or recall periods precluded assessment of joint occurrence of physical and nonphysical problems.

No systematic efforts have yet been made, in the conceptualization of child health status in the national health surveys, to put these various characteristics together in a composite profile or index of child health, or even to examine the relationships among the various components of health status. Since it is unlikely that health care reform would be expected to improve any of the specific components of health status as obtained in existing surveys, summary measures that would allow for the detection of changes in the composite of health characteristics would be more useful. Fortunately, researchers in child (as well as adult) health status are now developing methods that will make such an approach feasible (Starfield et al., 1992).

Monitoring health care reforms will also require more in-depth information on access to care, use of health services, and satisfaction with care than has previously been available in national surveys. The new Family Resources Supplement to the National Health Interview Survey represents a major step forward in this area. This module contains a number of useful questions on usual sources of care, characteristics of the source of care and caregiver, satisfaction with services, and delays in obtaining care. Since most reform efforts explicitly recognize that primary care is a central component, efforts to develop assessments of the adequacy of primary care will also be critically important. Although the Family Resource Supplement includes questions designed to distinguish primary care services from specialty care services, other national surveys do not. Therefore, the design and implementation of standardized methods to determine children's exposure to and experiences with primary care are of high priority.

Provider Surveys

Historically, survey data from practitioners and facilities have been used to provide information about the characteristics of hospitalizations and ambulatory care visits, primarily those to office-based physicians. New surveys sponsored by the National Center for Health Statistics have expanded the range of facilities and services studied to include ambulatory surgery centers, home and hospice care providers, and ambulatory care provided by hospitals. However, since the information obtained typically concerns individual encounters, it is not possible to link hospitalizations or visits made by individuals from one time to another or from one provider to another. Therefore, elucidation of differences in practice patterns is not possible. These types of data are primarily useful in providing information about the challenges of practice, e.g., information on the distribution and types of problems encountered in practices of different specialists, and a major contribution of such surveys, particularly the National Ambulatory Medical Care Survey, has been to elicit the nature of the problem, as perceived by the patient, that is responsible for initiating the visit. (However, the problem is generally recorded by the physician and thus may not accurately represent the problem just as the patient views it.) Refinements of these datasets so that they contain coded patient identifiers to enable linkages between events, and the encouragement of the use of coding systems to facilitate the analysis of patients' presenting problems and their relationships with the ensuing processes of care, will contribute in a major way to improving their utility for exploring differences in practice patterns, for clinical research, and for provider education.

Another concern pertains specifically to children. Due to limited funds, the sponsoring agency for datasets such as the National Ambulatory Medical Care Survey often makes use of supplementary funds provided by other agencies to enrich the dataset. Since these agencies generally heavily represent adult interests rather than those of children, data obtained from this and other surveys have generally contained more information about care provided for adult problems than for children's problems. Better balance between adult and children's interests is warranted as the era of health care reform emerges.

Administrative Records

Although there are some notable attempts to compile and use administrative data concerning the provision of health services (for example, the databases maintained by Systemetrics/Medstat and the United Health Care Corporation), there are some major problems in using existing administrative record data for health care reforms. One notable problem concerns the identification of the "denominator." Data are available for beneficiaries (i.e., those covered by health plans), but they exclude family members (often children) who are not covered. The identity of these nonbeneficiaries is generally unknown. Second, the most commonly used datasets are restricted to beneficiaries of corporate plans, and their generalizability to persons insured individually or in small groups is questionable. In other types of plans, ownership determines control over accessibility and dissemination of the data. Consequently, many administrative datasets are not available for surveillance of costs, access and quality. None of the administrative databases are currently able to provide adequate denominators, or to focus on per-capita total expenditures and utilization (rather than prices and individual claims—Gaus et al., 1993). Third, the completeness and quality of data are uneven as a result of unstandardized procedures for collecting them at the original source in health plans. Fourth, the data lack elements that would be critical in accomplishing the aims of health care reform. In particular, the data sources rarely contain information on presenting problems and baseline health status, against which improvements resulting from health services interventions could be judged.

The usefulness of existing administrative data is also compromised by inadequacies in current coding systems for ambulatory care diagnoses and problems. The International Classification of Diseases, which was developed primarily to code causes of death, is not well suited to classifying the problems in ambulatory care, especially in primary care, in which so many of the health problems cannot be resolved to formal diagnoses. Practitioners in many other countries have adopted the International Classification of Health Problems in Primary Care (ICHPPC) to facilitate the recording and analysis of information about the diagnoses that are managed in primary care, and the International Classification of Primary Care (ICPC) builds on the ICHPPC but adds the capability to code and classify presenting problems as well. To date, however, administrative databases in the United States have not attempted to adopt or adapt these primary-care-oriented classification systems.

The inadequacy of systems of classification and coding has been particularly problematic in the area of mental health problems. The development of the Diagnostic and Statistical Manual (DSM) has been a major advance for the practice of psychiatry, since it specifies criteria for the full range of diagnoses that occur in mental health services. It has not, however, been useful in primary care. Work currently under way will lead to the development of DSM-PC, an adaptation suitable for primary care. Companion efforts will also lead to the development of a version for children, which should be rapidly tested, promulgated, and considered for use, along with the ICPC, in clinical and administrative data.

Administrative data sources also lack information on the disposition of visits, particularly with regard to referrals for consultation (secondary care) and highly complex services (tertiary care). They also lack information on the type of professionals who deliver the services—information that is essential in understanding the appropriate roles for different types of primary care providers and specialists.

The adoption and promulgation of a national standardized ambulatory care minimum dataset, with carefully defined elements are long overdue. First proposed in 1980, such a dataset is still under discussion. Responsibility for its delayed adoption is due at least in part to controversies over the importance and necessity of certain data elements, issues concerning the confidentiality of data about individual patients, individual providers, and individual health care plans (which may regard such information as proprietary), and intensive lobbying by special-interest groups for inclusion of data elements of particular interest to them. Clearer specification of the goals of health care reform, with regard to its impact on effectiveness and efficiency of care, may help to specify those data elements that are most important.

Administrative databases frequently do not provide identifiers that enable the linkage of family members, and sometimes do not even contain identifiers that permit linkage of different health care events experienced by individuals. For example, hospital discharge data provide counts of hospitalizations and the characteristics associated with them, but they do not provide data on the number of individual people experiencing those hospitalizations or the characteristics of people who have more than one hospitalization.

Despite the many limitations in administrative data, the potential of these types of data for contributing to knowledge and policy is amply demonstrated by the data systems associated with the Medicare program. For example, it is now possible to link the Medicare Current Beneficiary Survey with Health Care Financing Administration claims payment files and with the National Death Index, Social Security records, and the Area Resource File (Wunderlich, 1992).

System Surveillance Data

The Area Resource File is the most commonly used source of information on system characteristics. It is a compilation of health-related data for each of the 3,070 counties in the country. Since the dataset contains census data on the size and characteristics of the population, rates can be calculated and compared over time and across areas. Data are derived from many sources, including the American Medical Association, the American Osteopathic Association, and the American Hospital Association; also included are data on health maintenance organizations in each county.

Health care reform is likely to pose additional challenges to system surveillance. Increasing formalization of health services delivery arrangements will make it possible and necessary to collect data on deployment of personnel by type and with regard to the characteristics of the populations served. Ensuring adequacy and equity of services will require attention to the balance between specialists and primary care practitioners in individual health plans; currently, such information is not available. Comparisons of health care risks, both for financial planning as well as for evaluation of effectiveness of care, in different populations will require improved case-mix measures applied in the same way in all areas.

Data sources such as the Area Resource File could be uniquely valuable in health care reform research by producing knowledge about the relationships between the structures, processes, and outcomes of health services and by exploring the trade-offs between access, quality, and costs of care. Since these types of data sources provide critical information about many aspects of the structure of services and some important aspects of health status at the population level, they can play an important role in efforts to understand the impact of system characteristics on provider practice characteristics, on people's use of services, and on the impact of health services on health outcomes and expenditures.

CONSIDERATIONS IN DESIGNING A STRATEGY FOR MONITORING CHANGES IN HEALTH CARE FOR CHILDREN AND FAMILIES

As demonstrated in the previous section, the nation possesses a rich set of vital statistics and surveillance data, survey data, administrative record data, and systems surveillance data that can serve as building blocks for a system to monitor health care reforms. Since these databases were not originally designed to monitor the performance of the health care system and its impact on health, modifications are needed. Below, we outline what we believe to be essential attributes of an effective system for monitoring health care reforms and summarize, in a general fashion, what changes need to be made to create a monitoring system with these attributes. The attributes include comprehensiveness, timeliness, ability to meet descriptive and analytical needs, ability to assess change, ability to measure short-term and long-term effects, provision of adequate geographic detail, capacity to assess effects on vulnerable populations, flexibility to address emerging issues, and capacity to integrate information within and across data bases.

Comprehensiveness

The framework presented in Table 1 suggests several domains of data needed for a comprehensive assessment of the impact of health care reforms on children and families. These domains include access, utilization, expenditures, health status, health resources, quality, and effectiveness of care. Existing data sets are generally designed to provide information on one or two of these domains, and in rare cases three or four. Consequently, assessing effects of reforms across multiple domains requires integrating databases (as discussed below). Since both public and private databases are needed to assess the effects of reform across these domains, a public-private partnership will be required.

The effects of health care reforms are also felt at multiple levels. At the population level, health care reforms affect individuals, families, and communities. Within the health care provider community, health care reforms have effects at the level of the individual practitioner or facility, the health plan level, and at the system level. In monitoring reforms, it is important to describe and document changes in each of these areas. However, existing databases (with the exception of systems surveillance data) are designed for the most part to provide information at the level of the individual patient or consumer. They are generally less suitable in their current form for assessing outcomes aggregated at the level of families, communities, and systems of care. Additional efforts will be required to assess outcomes at these aggregate levels. For example, there is a need for family-level identifiers in all household-based health surveys. In some surveys, such as the National Health Interview Survey, it is currently very difficult to identify records for parents of sample children, making family-level analysis all but impossible. Other surveys, such as the Current Population Survey, include family-level records and identifiers. Yet even in this dataset, it can be difficult to identify relationships among family members, especially in multigenerational households.

Much more work is required to assess effects at the community level. As a starting point, geographic identifiers are needed in national surveys to link systems surveillance data, such as that available in the Area Resource File, to population data. In the past, strict interpretation of confidentiality provisions have precluded such linkages. Although confidentiality must be respected, a review of policy in this area is called for.

Timeliness

In gauging the impact of health care reforms, policy makers, researchers, advocacy groups, and others will require timely information. Speedy acquisition, processing, and release of data are also essential if the monitoring system is to provide an early warning of problems or unintended consequences of reform. Hence, the implementation of reforms will increase pressure on sponsoring agencies to speed the collection, processing, and release of data. The pressure will be greatest for the larger, more complex survey efforts, such as the National Medical Expenditure Survey. This survey involves multiple personal interviews, diaries, and verification of expenditures through record checks. Partly as a consequence of the enormity of this undertaking, the 1977 and 1987 editions of this survey were largely outdated by the time processing was completed and data were released.

Trade-offs are always present between precision of data and production time. These competing needs must, of course, be balanced. One approach to addressing this issue is to develop a monitoring system that combines quick turnaround descriptive data for surveillance purposes with more precise but necessarily more slowly produced data for analytic and evaluative purposes. Taking this approach, data from large-scale population and provider surveys would be used for in-depth analysis and evaluation of health care reform. A complementary tracking system, based on rapid turnaround data sources, would be created to provide an early warning of problems and unintended consequences. The tracking system should be designed to provide rapid release information on a continuous basis as reform is implemented. Information for the tracking system could be derived from a combination of administrative data, public health surveillance data, and telephone survey data. Administrative data would be derived from health plans, claims payment systems and other sources. Public health surveillance data would come from existing and new surveillance efforts organized by the Centers for Disease Control and Prevention, as well as state and local public health agencies. Telephone surveys would provide immediate data on access barriers, satisfaction with care, and other indicators not available from administrative and public health surveillance systems. A capacity to conduct rapid turnaround telephone surveys is now being developed at the National Center for Health Statistics (NCHS, 1993). However, new funding would be required to implement such a program.

Meeting Descriptive and Analytical Needs

It is necessary for the monitoring system to provide information for both descriptive and analytical purposes. The objective of descriptive studies is *to describe* a phenomenon of interest, whereas the purpose of an analytical study is *to explain* the phenomenon (Aday, 1989; Moore, 1993). Descriptive data are needed to profile the status of children, families, and communities as well as providers and systems of care under health care reforms. Data are also needed for analytical purposes, such as unraveling relationships among variables or explaining trends. For example, the federal and state maternal and child health agencies may be interested in assessing whether and how patterns of care change for chronically ill children after health care reform is implemented. A descriptive profile of utilization patterns could be created from population and provider surveys and administrative records. If chronically ill children's utilization patterns were found to change substantially after implementation of reform, there would be a clear need to move beyond description of the changes to an explanation of whether the changes were caused by reforms or other factors, and which specific factors were responsible for them.

Data for both descriptive and analytical purposes are essential, but databases must be designed carefully if they are to meet both needs. Typically, more depth is needed within a topic area for analytical studies, whereas descriptive studies are often facilitated by fewer, carefully chosen measures. Hence, trade-offs can exist in meeting descriptive and analytical needs. One of the objectives in designing a monitoring system is balancing these needs.

Capacity to Assess Change

Assessment of change is fundamental to monitoring the impact of health care reform. Ideally, a monitoring system should have the capacity to provide information on changes occurring for children, families, and communities as well as providers and systems of care across multiple domains (access, utilization, expenditures, health status, health resources, quality, and effectiveness of care).

Two analytical approaches can be taken to measure change. First, data collected on a periodic basis can be analyzed and compared over time. For example, health insurance data from the Current Population Survey are frequently compared over time to assess changes in the number and proportion of uninsured persons. For such comparisons to be meaningful, at least certain items in the questionnaire must remain constant, since even small changes in questionnaire wording can have significant effects on survey responses. An example of this problem can be seen in the 1981 and 1988 Child Health Supplements to the National Health Interview Survey. Both supplements contained a checklist of child health conditions. Although the wording for many condition entries remained the same, the wording for others changed—precluding comparisons of prevalence over time. Although it is sometimes possible to estimate the impact of wording changes when questionnaires are changed, doing so is difficult and requires special attention.

The second approach consists of assessing changes over time within a panel of subjects (e.g., children, families, practitioners). In this case, the same subjects are followed with measures of interest collected at regular intervals. Panels can be created from samples obtained from vital statistics (e.g., birth records), administrative records (e.g., claims records), or survey samples. The panel approach is used most often in the survey context.

Although a powerful tool for assessing and analyzing change, panel surveys have been used only occasionally in child health. The most well-known panel surveys, including the Survey of Income and Program Participation and the National Longitudinal Survey of Youth, have limited health content. The few examples in the child health field include the National Survey of Family Growth and the National Maternal and Infant Health Survey, both sponsored by the National Center for Health Statistics. With the exception of these surveys, which have very specific purposes and limited target populations, there are no ongoing panel surveys of children's health.

Two promising possibilities for panel surveys are now being planned that could be of enormous value in monitoring health care reforms. First, the National Center for Health Statistics is considering conducting a child and family survey as part of the National Health Interview Survey. This comprehensive survey of child and family health would be modeled after the very successful 1988 National Health Interview Survey on Child Health. Like its predecessor, the new survey could collect in-depth information on pregnancy and birth, injuries, impairments, acute and chronic conditions, developmental and learning and behavioral problems, use of health services, and participation in health programs such as the Supplemental Food Program for Women, Infants, and Children, Medicaid, and Healthy Start. In addition, the planned survey would include several indicators of family functioning. If a panel or follow-up component was added, the survey could be an extremely valuable tool for assessing the effects of health care reforms on children and families. However, it is not clear at present whether even the baseline for this important survey will be fielded. The costs of this survey must be met externally by agencies interested in the survey results, and so far only limited funding has been committed. Unless additional funding becomes available soon, survey planning will be abandoned.

The second promising panel survey is the Survey of Program Dynamics, now being fielded by the Bureau of the Census. This survey includes a panel of 20,000 households first assembled in 1993 as part of the Survey of Income and Program Participation. The households will be followed over a 10-year period, with household interviews conducted annually or more frequently. As envisioned by its planners, the survey would focus on providing an information base for policy makers and researchers interested in welfare reform and health care reform issues. Initial funding has been provided by federal agencies interested in welfare reform, but so far no funding has been provided for the health care reform component.

Capacity to Measure Short- and Long-Term Effects

Health care reforms are likely to bring about a myriad of changes in the organization, financing, and delivery of care. Some of these changes will begin occurring during implementation or shortly after reforms are implemented; others will occur much later. For example, changes in access and utilization of care could be expected to occur soon after implementation of a reform. In contrast, changes in child health status, if they occur, are likely to become apparent only years later. Hence, the monitoring system must be capable of capturing changes occurring over the short and the long term.

As reforms are implemented at the state level, there are likely to be policy adjustments in eligibility, benefits, cost-sharing, and other components especially during the early years of reform and perhaps on an ongoing basis, if past experience with Medicaid and Medicare can serve as a guide. Consequently, the "effects" of reform are likely to change over time, as policy makers fine-tune various elements of the health care reform plan.

The monitoring system should then be designed with recognition of the temporal and ongoing nature of change. This means a monitoring system based on a simple "before and after" design will provide only partial and perhaps misleading conclusions concerning the effects of reform. Instead, the monitoring system should be conceived as an ongoing activity with continuous collection of outcome data.

Provision of Adequate Geographic Detail

Most major federal health data bases were originally designed to provide national or regional level estimates. State-level data will be critical in evaluating health care reforms, since reform is likely to be implemented differently in each state (and perhaps only in selected states). Indeed, as we've said, even without national health care reform, states are already beginning to implement their own reform agendas. Consequently, state-level data represent a key component of the monitoring system. All states maintain vital records and many maintain data collection systems for hospital discharge information. Claims payment systems are also maintained by every state Medicaid agency, although not all lend themselves to analysis. A few states have also developed household survey databases (Hawaii, Rhode Island, Puerto Rico), and all states participate in the behavioral risk factor surveys sponsored by the Centers for Disease Control and Prevention. However, no state currently has a data system in place that is capable of assessing the broad range of effects shown in Table 1. Moreover, none of the major federal health surveys currently has the capacity to assess the effects of state-level reform efforts on children and families.

Two survey design considerations are particularly relevant to producing state-level estimates from national surveys. First, the sample design, particularly the selection of primary sampling units, must be developed in a manner that is consistent with state-level estimation. In the past, major health surveys, such as the National Health Interview Survey, have selected primary sampling units that overlap state boundaries or have excluded some states entirely. This is now changing at least in some surveys. For example, the 1995 redesign of the National Health Interview Survey will include only primary sampling units that do not cross state boundaries, and all states will be represented for the first time. Second, there must be a sufficient number of cases at the state level to permit accurate estimation. Even in large household surveys, such as the National Health Interview Survey, there are insufficient numbers of observations in all but the largest states to permit useful state-level estimates. To a degree, this problem can be circumvented by combining multiple years of survey data. However, this strategy will have limited applicability to small states. Other approaches, such as supplementing household interviews with telephone interviews, need to be considered.

Over the long term, federal efforts should also be directed toward improving capacity at the state and local levels to conduct surveys, make better use of claims data and other administrative databases, and develop standards and conventions for sharing data between levels of government. The National Center for Health Statistics, with its long history of cooperating with states on the development of uniform standards for vital statistics, may be well suited to leading this effort.

With health care reforms in place, there will be a much greater need for coordinated information at the local, state, and national levels. As indicated earlier, data collection and retrieval need to be coordinated so that data collected at the local level can be aggregated to the state and federal level, and so that data collected at higher levels can be related to data collected at local levels. Doing so will permit comparison of effects across communities, states, and the nation.

Capacity to Assess Outcomes for Vulnerable Populations

The monitoring system should have a built-in capacity for assessing outcomes for vulnerable child populations, including children living in poor and near-poor families, minority children, children in out-of-home placements, and children with disabilities and other ongoing health problems.

These vulnerable populations are likely to be affected more significantly by health care reform than other populations. Consequently, there is a heightened need to closely monitor their welfare as reforms are implemented. Yet it is difficult to identify these children in vital records, administrative records, and public health surveillance systems. In surveys, sample sizes for these populations are often too limited for meaningful analysis. In the past, sample size problems have plagued analysis of health survey data for minority populations. During recent years, survey designers have improved capabilities in this area through oversampling of minority populations. For example, the National Health Interview Survey currently oversamples blacks and will begin oversampling Hispanics in 1995. However, difficulties remain in analyzing other vulnerable populations.

Two populations of particular concern are children residing in institutional settings and homeless children. Virtually all ongoing health surveys exclude children residing in institutions. Even the 1990 decennial census data on the institutionalized population lacks the specificity needed to estimate the number of children residing in institutions for health-related reasons. Even less information is available on homeless children and families. This population is routinely excluded from national household surveys and other data systems, even though local surveys have demonstrated significant unmet health needs exist for homeless children and families (Wood et al., 1990a, 1990b).

Emerging Issues

It is not possible to accurately predict the direction or timing of health care reform, or its effects, especially unintended consequences. As a result, flexibility in data collection will be necessary. During recent years, many ongoing surveys have adopted a modularized approach, whereby a core questionnaire is supplemented with modular questionnaires on topics of current interest. This provides an effective means for maintaining flexibility in data collection.

Unfortunately, the fielding of a "supplement" often depends on the availability of special funding for it. As a result, supplements generally reflect the interests of specific groups that have the resources to offer. For this reason, children have only infrequently been the subject of these added modules. To adequately monitor the effects of health care reform on children and families, an in-depth child and family supplement should be conducted at least every five years and preferably every three years as part of the National Health Interview Survey. Doing so would provide the flexibility needed to address emerging issues for children and families.

Integrating Data Collection Efforts

Over time, federal databases have become increasingly specialized and categorical in nature. The result is that few databases contain data across the multiple domains relevant to health care reform (access, utilization, expenditures, health status, health resources, effectiveness, and quality of care). Consequently, the monitoring system will be required to draw on multiple data sources. Its capacity for assessing the effects of reforms will be enhanced to the extent that data from the different databases can be integrated. Integrating or linking data from various sources offers the added advantage of increasing the utility of existing data bases at a relatively modest cost (AHCPR, 1991).

Integrating data can occur at several levels. At the most basic level, databases should share common definitions and terminology whenever possible; unfortunately, this happens less frequently than is desirable. For example, the National Health Interview Survey, the National Medical Expenditure Survey, the Current Population Survey, and the Survey of Income and Program Participation use different questions for assessing health insurance coverage. This makes it very difficult to compare results across surveys, or even to develop agreed-on estimates of the size of the insured and uninsured populations. Even commonly used terms such as *access* have imprecise meanings and varying representation in data collection efforts. The National Committee on Vital and Health Statistics should perhaps be given the responsibility for coordinating efforts to define important terms so that they can be measured in consistent ways.

Linking data across databases can yield significant benefits but presents additional challenges. Recently, much attention has been focused on linking administrative records such as claims payment data to national survey data. For example, data on utilization and expenditures from Medicare administrative files are linked to population-based survey data in the Medicare Current Beneficiary Survey. Similarly, the National Death Index now permits linkage of death certificates to most of the population surveys sponsored by the National Center for Health Statistics. The challenge ahead lies in integrating databases across federal agencies as well as between public and private data collection organizations.

Linkages of administrative data with survey data could provide a powerful mechanism to explore the relationship between services provided and resulting health status in the geographic area served by health services organizations and plans. Accomplishing this level of integration requires close cooperation among the sponsors of the databases. This has not always been possible in the past because of confidentiality issues, as well as concerns such as funding and turf. Health care reform will mean that new efforts toward integrating databases will be essential.

CONCLUSION

A carefully designed data collection and analysis strategy is central to assessing the impact of the changing health care system on children and families. In previous sections of this paper we presented a framework for assessing data needs, reviewed existing databases, and articulated the attributes of an effective monitoring system. All of this needs to be considered within an overall strategy for monitoring health care reforms. Too often data collection and analysis efforts are divorced, resulting in missed opportunities and inefficient use of resources. Data collection strategies must be developed in conjunction with a data analysis strategy. The data collection and analysis strategy should be driven by a clear understanding of the key health care reform issues. The specifics of that strategy and the monitoring system that will support it should be developed using a process that takes into account the needs and views of policy makers, the scientific community, child health advocates, and others concerned with the well-being of children.

The strategy of planning for data to monitor and assess changes in health care faces four types of challenges:

• *Concept development.* As the country moves toward primary care and toward outcome and functional status assessment, concerted attention will be needed to clarify the meaning of these concepts, especially as they relate to children, so that approaches to measurement can be developed.

• *Standardized measurement.* At present, the many different data systems and data sets use different criteria to measure the same concept. Important goals of health care reform, such as improving access and quality of care, are currently being measured in many different and incompatible ways. Once the concepts of access, quality, primary care, and health and functional status are clarified, attention must be devoted to developing consistent or at least compatible ways of measuring them.

• *Personal identifiers with maintenance of confidentiality.* Since person-focused (rather than disease-focused) health care requires the tracking of events over time and places for each individual in the population, a method of assigning unique personal identifiers that maintains confidentiality will need to be developed and instituted.

• *Responsibility and accountability.* Timely and accurate information is needed to ensure that changes consequent to health care reforms proceed in the anticipated direction.

In an ideal world, a system for monitoring health care reforms would be designed and implemented without regard to budget constraints. Realistically, limited additional funds are likely to be available for the monitoring system. Consequently, there is a need for careful consideration of the marginal costs and marginal benefits of adding components to the monitoring system. As much as possible, the system should rely on existing data bases, modifying them when necessary but keeping in mind their original purposes. Fortunately, the nation already possesses a rich set of health databases that can be used for monitoring health care reforms. With careful planning and coordination, the vast number of current surveys might even be reduced, thus releasing resources that could better be applied to obtaining data of better quality with more rapid availability. Such planning will be required to develop a system capable of accurately and economically assessing the effects of health care reform in a timely fashion.

REFERENCES

Aday, L.
1989 *Designing and Conducting Health Surveys.* San Francisco: Jossey-Bass Inc.

Agency for Health Care Policy and Research (AHCPR)
1991 *Report to Congress: The Feasibility of Linking Research-Related Data Bases to Federal and Non-Federal Medical Administrative Data Bases.* AHCPR Pub. No. 91-0003. Rockville, Md.: AHCPR.

Benson, V., and M.A. Marano
1994 *Current Estimates from the National Health Interview Survey*. Vital Health Statistics, Series 10, Number 189. Hyattsville, Md.: National Center for Health Statistics.

Edwards ,W.S., D.M. Winn, and V. Kurlantzick et al.
1994 Evaluation of National Health Interview Survey Diagnostic Reporting. *Vital Health Statistics*, Series 2, Number 120. National Center for Health Statistics.

Fox, H.B., and M.A. McManus
1992 *Medicaid Managed Care Arrangements and Their Impact on Children and Adolescents: A Briefing Report*. Washington, D.C.: Fox Health Policy Consultants.

Gaus, C., J. Scanlon, and M. Ross
1993 A New Information Framework for Health Care Reform. Presented at the Annual Meeting of National Association of Health Data Organizations, Washington, D.C., December 9.

Jameson, E., and E. Wehr
1993 Drafting national health care reform legislation to protect the health interests of children. *Stanford Law and Policy Review Journal* 5(Fall):1.

Lamberts, H., and M. Wood, eds.
1987 *International Classification of Primary Care*. World Health Organization of National Colleges, Academies, and Academic Associations of General Practitioners/Family Physicians. Oxford: Oxford University Press.

Leginski, W., C. Goze, F. Driggers, S. Dupman, D. Geersten, E. Kamis-Gould, M. Namerow, R. Patton, N. Wilson, and C. Worster
1989 *Data Standards for Mental Health Decision Support System*. DHHS Pub. No. (Adm) 89-1589, FN-10. Washington, D.C.: U.S. Department of Health and Human Services.

Moore, K.
1993 Children and Families: Data Needs in the Next Decade. Presented at the interagency Family Data Working Group meeting, Washington, D.C., May 25.

National Center for Health Statistics, Centers for Disease Control and Prevention
1993 *Surveys for Monitoring Health Reform*. Presented at the AHSR/FHSR annual meeting, June 27-29.

Newacheck, P., D.C. Hughes, J.J. Stoddard, N. Halfon
1994 Children with chronic illness and Medicaid managed care. *Pediatrics* 93(3):497-500 (Commentary).

Snider, S., and S. Boyce
1994 *Sources of Health Insurance and Characteristics of the Uninsured: Analysis of the March 1993 Current Population Survey*. EBRI Issue Brief Number 145. Washington, D.C.: Employee Benefit Research Institute.

Starfield, B.
1973 Health services research: a working model. *New England Journal of Medicine* 289:132-136.
1992 *Primary Care: Concept, Evaluation, and Policy*. New York: Oxford University Press.

Wood, D.L., R.B. Valdez, T. Hayashi, and A. Shen
1990a Homeless and housed families in Los Angeles: a study comparing demographic, economic and family function characteristics. *American Journal of Public Health* 80:1049-1053.
1990b A study comparing the health of homeless children and housed, poor children. *Pediatrics* 86:858-866.

World Organization of National Colleges, Academies, and Academic Associations of General Practitioners/Family Physicians (WONCA)

1979 *International Classification of Health Problems in Primary Care.* ICHPPC-2, 2nd Ed., Oxford: Oxford University Press.

Wunderlich, G., ed.

1992 *Toward A National Health Care Survey.* Panel on the National Health Care Survey, Committee on National Statistics, National Research Council. Washington, D.C.: National Academy Press.

Estimating the Incidence, Causes, and Consequences of Interpersonal Violence for Children and Families

Colin Loftin and James A. Mercy

Accurate data for estimating the incidence, causes, and consequences of violence for children and families are critical to developing effective policies and programs for prevention and control of violence. Currently, however, federal data collection activities only incidentally address key data needs, and methodology is not sufficiently consistent to provide a solid underpinning for policy and program development. In this paper, we describe the current data collection system and assess the need for improvement.

The paper is limited to data collection focused on serious assaultive violence in primary relationships, such as families, and violence involving children. As a general concept, *violence* is broad, including any use of force or threats of force regardless of intent or magnitude. Accordingly, it includes an argument in which threats were exchanged, spanking, and vicious, lethal rape.

A hypothetical J-shaped distribution of the magnitude of harm from violent behavior reveals opposite problems in trying to estimate the incidence of violent behavior (Figure 1). On the left side of the curve, the

Colin Loftin is director of the Violence Research Group, Department of Criminology and Criminal Justice, University of Maryland. James A. Mercy is with the Division of Violence Prevention, National Center for Injury Prevention and Control, Centers for Disease Control and Prevention.

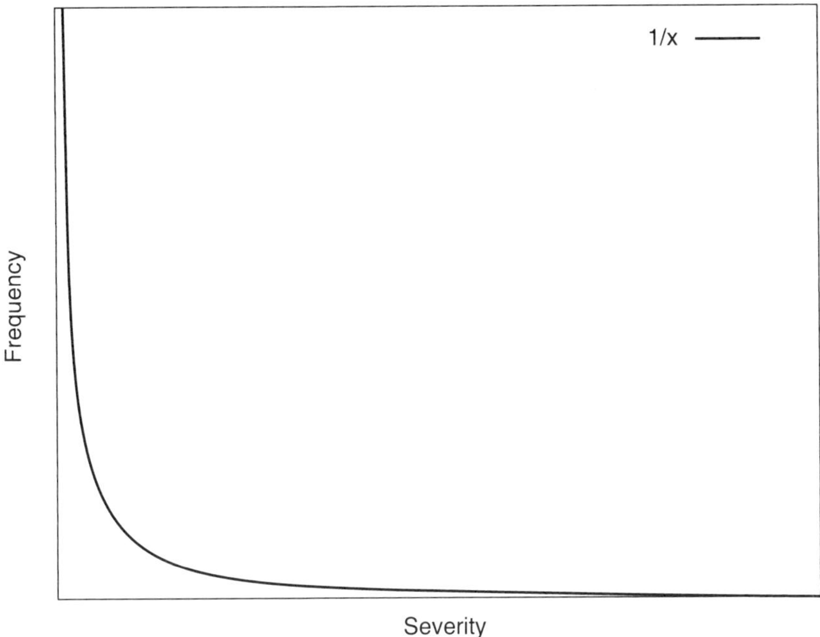

FIGURE 1 Hypothetical Relationship Between Frequency and Severity

incidents are so frequent and so inconsequential that they should not, and probably cannot, be estimated. On the right side, the events are so rare that they will be missed by standard sampling schemes, yet they are so harmful that they are of major concern.

Without specifying an exact cutoff, we are primarily interested in the right half of the distribution. It includes violent behavior that results in physical injury, as well as other intentional acts that pose a significant risk of injury. A wide range of extremely harmful incidents are omitted from consideration. We do not deal with negligence or failure to act that may result in injury; psychological trauma, if there is no threat of force; or self-directed violence, such as suicide or suicide attempts.

We begin by describing major approaches to collecting information on serious assaultive violence and characterizing their methodology, without attempting an exhaustive description of all of the major data collection systems. We then describe what we see as some of the major problems and pressing needs. The paper ends by suggesting some feasible approaches to addressing these needs.

EXISTING DATA COLLECTION SYSTEMS AND APPROACHES

Approaches to collecting data on serious assaultive violence can be divided according to the general sampling strategies used. Household surveys sample dwelling units and obtain self-reports of offending and/or victimization from persons residing in those dwellings. Organization-based surveys sample service providers such as schools, social agencies, and emergency departments and obtain information from either self-reports or records. Complete enumerations or registries, such as the National Center for Health Statistics' vital statistics or the Federal Bureau of Investigation's Uniform Crime Reporting system, attempt to capture all of the incidents that occur in a target population. The fourth approach combines several sampling strategies and is used when the incidents being studied are infrequent and no single sampling frame would yield valid estimates. The sections that follow briefly describe some examples of each approach. The characteristics of the major data sources are also described in Table 1.

Household Surveys

The National Crime Victimization Survey, the National Youth Survey, and the National Family Violence Surveys are based on household samples. There are, of course, major methodological differences in the these surveys, but they provide useful illustrations of this approach.

The National Crime Victimization Survey

The National Crime Victimization Survey (NCVS, previously known as the National Crime Panel and the National Crime Survey) is a large, continuous survey of people at least 12 years old who live in U.S. residential housing units. The survey is conducted by the Bureau of the Census for the Bureau of Justice Statistics to provide national estimates of the incidence of criminal victimization (Bureau of Justice Statistics, 1992). Respondents are interviewed in person and by telephone seven times at 6-month intervals in a rotating panel design. Considerable attention is given to placing reported incidents in a specific time frame. For example, the first interview in a panel is used strictly for bounding (marking the beginning of the reference period for the second interview); thereafter, respondents are asked for the specific month of occurrence for each incident they report. NCVS data have been collected continuously since 1973 and include reports of victimizations that may not have been reported to the police.

The most distinctive feature of the NCVS is the extensive screening for crime incidents and the completion of separate incident forms that record specific information about each incident, including the exact month of occurrence, the victim-offender relationship, and the extent of injury and property loss.

The National Youth Survey

The National Youth Survey (NYS) is a longitudinal study of a national probability sample, selected in 1976, of 1,725 youths ages 11 to 17. The first interviews were conducted in 1977. By late 1993, nine waves of data had been collected (Elliott, 1994). The interview schedule contains, along with a variety of other measures, a set of self-reported delinquency items, and in some of the waves follow-up questions are designed to obtain some details about circumstances associated with the offense. Of particular interest are items designed to measure "serious violent offenses," defined as aggravated assault, robbery, and rape (Elliott, 1994:3):

- "[Have] you attacked someone with the idea of seriously hurting or killing that person?"
- "[Have] you used force or strong-arm methods to get money or things from people?"
- "[Have] you had or tried to have sexual relations with someone against their will?"

The measure of serious violent offenses is restricted to assaults, robberies, and rapes that involved "some injury or a weapon." Medically treated incidents are defined as those in which the victim was "cut or bleeding, had broken bones/jaw/nose, was unconscious, was taken to a hospital, or died" (Elliott, 1994:4). The survey also collects data on violent victimization of respondents.

National Family Violence Surveys

The National Family Violence Surveys were conducted in 1975 and 1985 (Straus et al., 1980; Gelles and Straus, 1988; Straus and Gelles, 1990). The 1975 survey was a national probability sample of 2,143 "currently married or cohabiting persons aged 18 through 70," stratified by region and demographic characteristics. Response Analysis Corporation conducted the hour-long personal interviews. A random half of respondents were women and if there was more than one child, the "referent child" was randomly selected from the children between ages 3 and 17 who resided in the household. The completion rate for the entire sample was 65 percent.

The 1985 survey, conducted by Louis Harris & Associates by telephone, included 6,002 households consisting of two married or cohabiting adults or an adult age 18 or older who had either divorced or separated within the last two years or a single parent living with a child under age 18.

TABLE 1 Major Data Sources for Measuring Interpersonal Violence

Data Collection	Target Population	Source of Data	Frequency of Collection	Violent Behavior	Sponsoring Organization
			Household Surveys		
National Crime Victimization Survey (NCVS)	Persons ≥ age 12	Mixed, personal and telephone interviews	Monthly	Rape, robbery, assault	Bureau of Justice Statistics (BJS)
National Youth Survey (NYS)	Persons ages 11-17 in 1976	Personal interviews	9 wave panel, 1977, 78, 79, 80, 81, 84, 87, 89, 93	Assault, robbery, rape	Collaboration: Violence and Traumatic Stress Branch, National Institute of Mental Health (NIMH) and Justice Department
National Family Violence Surveys	1975: Married and cohabiting persons ages 18-70 1985: Adult couples, recently separated persons, or single parents living in telephone households	1975: Personal interviews 1985: Telephone interviews	2 cross-sections, 1975 and 1985	Assaults (partners and children)	Violence and Traumatic Stress Branch, NIMH
National Survey of Families and Households (NSFH)	Persons ≥ age 19 living in households and able to be interviewed in either English or Spanish	Mixed, personal interviews and self-administered questionnaire	2-wave panel, 1987-1988 1992-1994	Hitting, shoving, and throwing things; injury in fight with partner	Center for Population Research, National Institute for Child Health and Human Development (NICHD)

National Survey of Children (NSC)	Households with at least one child (age 7-11 in 1976)	Personal interviews	Multiwave panel, 1976, 81, 87	Involuntary sexual intercourse	Multiple funding: Foundation for Child Development, Center for Population Research (NICHD) and others
National Women's Study (NWS)	Women ≥ age 18 living in telephone households	Telephone interviews	3-wave panel, 1989, 90, 91	Assault, rape	National Institute of Drug Abuse
Youth Risk Behavior Surveillance System: National Household-Based Surveys, National Health Interview Survey, Youth Risk Behavior Supplement (NHIS-YRBS)	Household population ages 12-21	Personal interviews and self-administered audiocassette questionnaire	Cross-section; follow-back of 1992 NHIS	Physical fights, fights with injury, who fought, weapon carrying	Collaboration: Centers for Disease Control and Prevention (CDC) and others
Organization-Based Surveys					
Youth Risk Behavior Surveillance System: National School-Based Surveys	Students in grades 9-12 in the 50 states, the District of Columbia, Puerto Rico, and the Virgin Islands	Self-administered questionnaires	Cross-section; biennial, odd-years	Physical fights, fights with injury, who fought, weapon carrying	Center for Chronic Disease Prevention and Health Promotion, CDC

continued on next page

TABLE 1 Continued

Data Collection	Target Population	Source of Data	Frequency of Collection	Violent Behavior	Sponsoring Organization
		Organization-Based Surveys (continued)			
Youth Risk Behavior Surveillance System: State and Local School-Based Surveys	Student in grades 9-12 in participating state or city	Self-administered questionnaires	Cross-section; participation varies with jurisdiction	Same as above, but may be modified in some jurisdictions	Collaboration between CDC and state local depts. of health and education
Monitoring the Future	High school seniors	Self-administered questionnaires	Annual since 1976	Assault	National Institute on Drug Abuse
National Electronic Injury Surveillance System (NEISS)	Nonfatal injuries treated in emergency departments	Medical records supplemented with telephone interviews with victims and witnesses	Monthly	Intentional injuries	Consumer Product Safety Commission, BJS and CDC
National Hospital Ambulatory Medical Care Survey (NHAMCS)	Patient visits to emergency and/or outpatient departments in nonfederal, short-stay hospitals	Medical records	Began December 1991	Intentional injuries	National Center for Health Statistics, CDC

Study of the National Incidence and Prevalence of Child Abuse and Neglect (NIS-I and II)	Children (< age 18) referred to community professionals	Forms completed by community agencies	2 cross-sections 1979-80 and 1986	Abuse and neglect	National Center on Child Abuse and Neglect
		Complete Enumerations			
Uniform Crime Reporting Program: Return A	Index crimes known to law enforcement agencies[a]	Police reports	Monthly	Murder[b], robbery, rape, assault	Federal Bureau of Investigation
Uniform Crime Reporting Program: Supplementary Homicide Report	Homicides that occurred in the U.S.	Police reports	Monthly	Homicide[c]	Federal Bureau of Investigation
Uniform Crime Reporting Program: Age, Sex, Race, and Ethnic Origin of Persons Arrested	Arrests for specified violent crimes	Police reports	Monthly	Arrests for violent crimes	Federal Bureau of Investigation
National Vital Statistics Mortality Data	Deaths due to intentional injuries	Death certificates	Exact time of death	Homicide	National Center for Health Statistics, CDC

continued on next page

TABLE 1 Continued

Data Collection	Target Population	Source of Data	Frequency of Collection	Violent Behavior	Sponsoring Organization
			Combined Strategies		
National Incidence Studies of Missing, Abducted, Runaway and Thrownaway Children	Children (< age 18)	Multiple modes of data collection	Cross-section, 1988	Abductions by strangers and nonfamily members	Office of Juvenile Justice and Delinquency Prevention

[a]Violent index crimes are murder and nonnegligent manslaughter, forcible rape, robbery, and aggravated assault.
[b]Includes nonnegligent manslaughter.
[c]Includes justifiable homicides as well as murders.

Within the household, eligible respondents and a referent child were selected randomly. Black and Hispanic households were oversampled, but the entire sample is weighted to be representative of the total U.S. population. The 1985 survey had a higher completion rate (85 percent) than did the 1975 survey, and interviews were administered in less time (35 minutes) (Straus and Gelles, 1990: 529-532).

Both surveys employed the conflict tactics scale (CTS), a set of questions about how interpersonal conflicts are resolved that is designed to allow respondents to report violence directed at household members with less response error than would alternative approaches. The CTS is not exactly a self-report, however, because respondents provide proxy information about their behavior and the behavior of other members of the household. As would be expected, the proxy responses have different characteristics than the self-reports.

Other Surveys

Other important household surveys on violent behaviors include the National Survey of Families and Households (Sweet et al., 1988; Brush, 1990); the National Survey of Children (Moore et al., 1989); and the National Women's Study (National Victim Center, 1992).

Organization-Based Surveys

Another strategy is to sample organizations such as schools, hospitals, police departments, and other agencies that provide services to victims and offenders. Prominent examples are school-based surveys of delinquent behavior such as Monitoring the Future and the school-based Youth Risk Behavior Surveys and hospital-based surveys of injuries such as the National Electronic Injury Surveillance System and the National Hospital Ambulatory Medical Care Survey (McCaig, 1994). Another important organization-based study that measures violence among families and children is the Study of the National Incidence and Prevalence of Child Abuse and Neglect, also called the National Incidence Study (National Center on Child Abuse and Neglect, 1988).

The main advantage of organization-based studies is that the per-case cost is lower than in household samples. This is certainly the case with school-based samples and samples of emergency departments, since one would have to screen hundreds of households to obtain a single case of assault or rape with serious physical injury.

Monitoring the Future

The Monitoring the Future studies are national multistage probability samples of senior classes in approximately 130 high schools. These studies have been conducted since about 1975 by the Survey Research Center at the University of Michigan. Among the self-report delinquency behaviors respondents are asked how many times during the previous 12 months they have (Osgood et al., 1989: 417):

- "Hit an instructor or supervisor"
- "Taken part in a fight where a group of your friends were against another group"
- "Hurt someone badly enough to need bandages or a doctor"
- "Used a knife of gun or some other thing (like a club) to get something from a person."

National Electronic Injury Surveillance System

The National Electronic Injury Surveillance System (NEISS) is designed to produce national estimates of the frequency and severity of injuries associated with specific consumer products. The system, which uses a stratified probability sample of hospital emergency departments in the United States and its territories, is conducted for the U.S. Consumer Product Safety Commission. Data are entered into the NEISS computer system from patient records each day; approximately 200,000 injury reports are collected through NEISS each year. Of these, about 1 percent are selected for follow-up investigation (case selection is dependent on the commission's product-specific priorities). Telephone interviews with victims or witnesses are then conducted to gather further information on events surrounding the injury incidents (U.S. Consumer Product Safety Commission, 1986). The Centers for Disease Control and Prevention and the Bureau of Justice Statistics are currently exploring the use of the NEISS system to collect information on injuries due to violence.

Complete Enumerations or Registries

There are two major systems that attempt to completely enumerate specified classes of assaultive violence: the Federal Bureau of Investigation's Uniform Crime Reporting System and the homicide portion of the mortality data from the vital statistics maintained by the National Center for Health Statistics.

These national enumeration systems serve two unique roles. First, they provide information on rare incidents such as homicide in specific groups (e.g., infants and spouses) (Fingerhut and Kleinman, 1989a, 1989b; Mercy and Saltzman, 1989). Second, they provide the basis for state and local estimates. Their value is limited, however, by the fact that little information is collected and data on individuals are collected only for deaths. Also, in the case of UCR data, there has been very little research on the quality of the records, and the research that has been done suggests serious problems (Loftin, 1986; Loftin et al., 1987; Rokaw et al., 1990).

Uniform Crime Reporting Program

The Uniform Crime Reporting (UCR) program of the Federal Bureau of Investigation compiles information on crimes reported to or discovered by local and state police agencies in the United States. The program attempts to account, in a consistent manner, for the amount of crime known to police across the country, despite jurisdictional variation in legal definitions and practices. In concept, all crimes that come to the attention of law enforcement and are classifiable as UCR incidents are reported through the UCR data collection system.

The main data collection instrument in the UCR is a form called "Return A": a police agency's monthly summary of recorded murders, rapes, robberies, burglaries, larcenies, auto thefts, and arsons. Other data forms submitted to the UCR program include the "Supplementary Homicide Report" (SHR), the "Supplement to Return A," "Law Enforcement Officers Killed and Assaulted," and "Age, Sex, Race, and Ethnic Origin of Persons Arrested" (Federal Bureau of Investigation, 1984). All of these except the SHR are summary reports that represent a monthly tally of various items requested by the UCR program. The SHR, in contrast, collects characteristics on each individual homicide incident investigated by the agency. The National Incident-Based Reporting System, which is under development, will provide incident-level information on all reportable offenses, but the system is currently implemented in only a few test jurisdictions (Poggio et al., 1985; Federal Bureau of Investigation, 1993:3).

With the exception of the SHR and the systems that are under development, the only data that identify age, race, and gender of offenders or victims are the arrest data. Therefore, the UCR data are of very limited value in studying violence in specific populations, such as families and children.

National Vital Statistics Mortality Data

Death certificates provide the basis of the national mortality data compiled by the Division of Vital Statistics of the National Center for Health Statistics (NCHS). Registration of births and deaths is a legal requirement in all states, and elements of the U.S. Standard Death Certificate, including such items as age, sex, race, place of residence, and place and cause of death, are recorded and forwarded to NCHS through state vital statistics records offices. Codes for cause of death, including those for homicide, are assigned according to definitions established by the *International Classification of Diseases, Ninth Revision* (World Health Organization, 1977).

Combined Strategies

The last type of design is actually a hybrid of approaches that draws on several sampling strategies to produce the estimates of interest. This design is motivated by the infrequency of the target incidents and the weaknesses of any single sampling frame to yield valid estimates of its incidence.

The National Incidence Studies of Missing, Abducted, Runaway and Thrownaway Children (NISMART) is a good example of a combined system. NISMART collects data from six separate sources: a household survey, a survey of juvenile facilities, interviews with returned runaways, police records, FBI data, and a survey of community professionals (Finkelhor et al., 1992). Although the focus of NISMART is on numbers of children and not on numbers of incidents per se, the design is instructive nonetheless.

The use of multiple methods and sources of data by NISMART investigators was partially dictated by a wide-ranging charge to examine the "missing children problem," one that they concluded was a set of at least five different and distinct problems (i.e., family abductions, nonfamily abductions, runaways, thrownaways, and lost or otherwise missing children). Examining even a single area, for example, nonfamily abductions, NISMART demonstrates the desirability of a combined approach. Although its large-scale telephone survey could generate sufficient cases to estimate the number of attempted abductions (albeit with a large standard error), it was not effective in estimating completed abductions, an apparently much rarer event. For these, the NISMART police records study proved a better approach (Finkelhor et al., 1992).

AREAS OF PRESSING NEED

Existing data on violent behavior and its influence on children and families are fragmented, variable in quality, and do not allow for addressing many important policy issues. In this section we identify areas of the most pressing need.

Obtaining Valid Responses

Asking respondents to report on complex, sensitive, traumatic, and even illegal behavior committed by themselves or by members of their household approaches the limits of what one can reasonably expect from survey methods. Estimates based on different methodologies vary considerably and result in confusion and even loss of confidence in the statistical estimates of violent behavior.

A couple of examples illustrate the point. A recent paper based on the National Youth Survey estimates that 36 percent of African-American males and 25 percent of non-Hispanic white males report having committed at least one aggravated assault, robbery, or rape during their 17th year, the peak year for offending (Elliott, 1994). This figure is surprisingly high and several times higher than estimates based on such sources as arrests and the reports of victims.

Similarly, the National Woman's Study estimates that, during 1990, 683,000 women age 18 or older were the victims of rape (National Victim Center, 1992: 2-3). This is more than five times the 1990 estimate based on the NCVS for people age 12 and older (Bureau of Justice Statistics, 1992: 5). Research is clearly needed in two general methodological areas: (1) eliciting candid responses about sensitive and traumatic incidents and (2) capturing the complexity of violent events.

Eliciting Candid Responses

Substantial research exists on enhancing the validity of responses about sensitive and illegal behaviors, such as sexual activities and drug use. Many of these existing techniques could be profitably applied to measuring violence. Special problems arise, however, in household interviews in which one member of the household is reported to have abused another. Reporting violent behavior may put respondents at greater risk of victimization and thus creates serious problems for data collection. This issue is of central importance because these are exactly the situations that have high incidence rates and a substantial influence on statistical estimates.

Capturing Complexity

Few existing data collection mechanisms capture much of the complexity of violent incidents. The experience in the NCVS with series victimization is one of many examples that might be cited. Many respondents are unable to recall the details of separate incidents, even with bounded interviews and relatively short reference periods, because there are so many similar assaults during a short period that they cannot remember them as separate incidents. These "series incidents" have been characterized as incidents with long duration rather than as individual events by Biderman (1981: 795). Counting them requires special methods. Although this issue is an essential feature of the underlying phenomenon, NCVS is the only survey that has confronted it.

Other features of violent incidents that should be captured are the severity of injuries and the extent of the other harmful effects of violence. This information is important not only for estimating the impact of violence on society, but also for defining incidents and comparing across data collection systems. Measures of self-reported offending would profit from some of the methodology that NCVS has developed for measuring victimization. Bounding interviews, using shorter reference periods, and requiring respondents to provide details of specific incidents would contribute important information about the nature of violence and, other things being equal, would increase the precision of estimates.

Undercoverage in Data Collection Systems on Violence

Undercoverage is another problem in violence data collection systems. People who are at high risk for violence, either as offenders or as victims, are also likely to be missed in surveys of households and schools. Again, a couple of examples illustrate the point.

Using evidence from police reports and an estimate of the case-fatality rate for gunshot wounds, Cook (1985) estimates that the number of nonfatal gunshot wounds is three times higher than the NCVS estimate. Although some of the difference may be due to the quality of police data, it is likely that many of the victims of gunshot wounds are not captured in household surveys.

The groups that are likely to be missed in household surveys—blacks, Hispanics, and other minorities; children under the age of 10; the poor; renters; and people who move frequently (Hogan, 1993; Robinston et al., 1993)—are also those at high risk for being victims or offenders. Those who are at highest risk and who may contribute disproportionately to incidence estimates are the ones most likely to be missed. This problem in coverage is especially true for children and adults who are part of several households or who otherwise live in nontraditional family settings.

Data on Risk Factors, Social Context, Consequences, and Sequences

Existing data collection systems on violence, particularly those that focus on the more severe forms of violence, are designed primarily for estimating the incidence of violent events. They do not collect very much information on risk factors, social contexts, and other covariates of violence that might be used in evaluating causal models. Systems would be considerably more valuable if they measured both incidence and important covariates.

It is ironic that the data collection systems that have the best information about the most serious violent incidents (such as the vital statistics mortality data and the NCVS) provide the least information about covariates, whereas those with a lot of information about covariates (such as the National Survey of Youth and the National Family Violence Surveys) provide little information about the most serious violent incidents.

Data on Precursors and Long-Term Consequences of Severe Assault

Violent assaults and deaths have major consequences for both primary and secondary victims (i.e., children, families, and friends of primary victims), but very little is known about the magnitude and long-term pattern of those consequences. Registration systems such as vital statistics mortality data or the files of law enforcement agencies contain virtually no information about precursors or the long-term consequences of violence. Surveys provide more information, but are still quite limited. The value of existing information could be magnified severalfold by sampling cases from the registration systems and interviewing victims or next of kin to obtain information about the consequences of victimization. Topics of study would include such items as long-term medical costs, disabilities, restricted activity, loss of time from work, impairment, and other circumstances surrounding violent incidents and lifestyles. Case-control studies comparing cases in the registration systems with controls and prospective studies following a group of victims and an appropriate control group of nonvictims would be valuable.

State and Local Estimates of the Incidence of Serious Assaultive Violence

Many of the programs and policies designed to prevent violence or mitigate its consequences are implemented at state and local levels, and evaluating the impact of these efforts is critical. Unfortunately, few data collection systems are capable of producing small-area estimates of serious assaultive violence. Of the major data collection systems, only the vital statistics mortality data and the UCR system can produce estimates for state and local areas, and there are major limitations in the value of these systems.

The vital statistics mortality data provide only a limited amount of information about victims besides age, race, gender, marital status, place of residence, and cause of death; there are no data about circumstances. A revision of the U.S. Standard Death Certificate, offered for state use beginning in 1989, included new items on the decedent's educational attainment and on Hispanic origin and expanded fields for indicating multiple or underlying causes of death (National Center for Health Statistics, 1993). For some states, "usual occupation" and "kind of business or industry" are also recorded.

In addition to limited numbers of variables, confidentiality concerns affect the availability of some types of information in the public-use data. Estimates for small areas are particularly affected. Since 1982, the mortality detail files have identified the decedent's county or city of residence only if the population was 100,000 or greater. Confidentiality restrictions also prevent aggregation of daily time series after 1987 from the public microdata because exact day of death is masked.

Data from the FBI's Supplementary Homicide Report provide information about both victims and offenders for state and local areas, but there are major coverage errors (whole states are missing in some years) and content errors (Loftin, 1986; Loftin et al., 1987).

STRATEGIES FOR IMPROVEMENT

Coordinate Federal Focus on Data Related to Violence

Chief among the strategies needed to improve data collection on violence involving children and families is the need to better coordinate and integrate federal efforts to collect, analyze, and disseminate such data. There is a growing interest in the problem of violence at the federal level, and numerous departments and agencies have overlapping interests in ensuring the availability and use of high-quality data. This coordination should extend beyond intradepartmental efforts to go across departments, such as health and human services, justice, education, labor, and housing and urban development.

The benefits of better coordination and integration are clear. First, pooling financial support for surveys and other data collection activities will allow more efficient use of limited resources. For example, the National Center for Injury Prevention and Control of the Centers for Disease Control and Prevention and the Bureau of Justice Statistics are currently working more or less independently to collect information on intentional injuries through the National Electronic Injury Surveillance System (described above). In addition, the National Institute for Occupational Safety and Health of the Centers for Disease Control and Prevention is interested in using these data for monitoring work-related violent injuries. This is a clear instance in which coordination and integration could improve data quality and increase efficiency in the use of federal resources.

Second, more consistent estimates of the incidence and prevalence of violence and related behaviors could be produced through the use of consistent definitions and methodologies for data collection across federal departments. The violence field, particularly in the realm of family violence, is rife with conflicting estimates of magnitude and trends. Coordinating definitions and methodologies could help improve the consistency in results across federal surveys.

A mechanism is needed to achieve meaningful coordination and integration. The Federal Forum on Aging Statistics, which has been instrumental in this process across the National Institute on Aging, the National Center for Health Statistics, and the Bureau of the Census, is a potential model. An interagency committee or a third party (such as the Committee on National Statistics) could also be useful.

Coordinated Methodological Research Program

Because the methodological problems of measuring violence and its impact on families and children are interrelated and similar across data collection systems, coordinated research on basic methodology would be appropriate. A consortium of agencies or the National Science Foundation could study issues such as:

- the relative effectiveness of different methods of screening for and measuring the characteristics of violent behavior, especially involving children and within households,
- the effects of alternative collection methods that protect respondents' privacy in household surveys,
- techniques for improving coverage of persons at high risk for personal violence in household surveys, and
- estimation procedures that incorporate information from multiple sampling frames, such as household samples and the records of service organizations.

Explore More Efficient Ways of Identifying Cases

Household surveys of serious assaultive violence require large, expensive screening operations because most of the households contacted will not have experienced a target incident. As a result, most of the expense of data collection is devoted to interviews that are not directly useful for analysis. Any procedure that increases the efficiency of screening will vastly improve the cost-effectiveness of surveys.

Two promising approaches to reducing the costs of screening are using multipurpose screening surveys and surveys that use both household samples and samples drawn from administrative records and registration systems. With multipurpose screening, a survey designed to locate children for a study of immunization could, for example, also locate them for a study of violent behavior. The same survey could also be used to locate older respondents for a study of elder abuse and other issues concerning older citizens.

Household samples and samples from administrative records are complementary and used together, as in the National Incidence Studies of Missing, Abducted, Runaway, and Thrownaway Children, provide a much broader range of data than they do separately.

Explore the Feasibility of Collecting Data in Key Health Care Settings

Changes in the way services are delivered provide opportunities for new data sources. Two changes in the health care system have already led to more accurate and informative data collection on violence. First, the growing movement to ensure that health care providers are sensitive to evidence that their patients are being abused has led to widespread training programs for health care students and practitioners and to protocols for identifying, assessing, and referring victims of violence. This advance has the potential of greatly improving the quality and depth of data that might be collected on violence from health care providers.

Second, the rising costs of health care in recent decades have spawned the development of health maintenance organizations, which, as health care reform evolves, are likely to provide primary health care to an increasingly larger proportion of the population. These organizations may be excellent sites for acquiring data on the incidence of violence, particularly family and intimate violence, in defined populations and on the health consequences of violence and its impact on child and family development. We need to explore the feasibility of developing and testing alternative methods for data collection in health maintenance organizations and other key health care settings (e.g., emergency departments, public prenatal clinics).

Develop Efficient Ways for Small-Area Estimation

State and local data provide a crucial underpinning for developing and evaluating local prevention policies and programs because patterns of violence differ across regions and localities. For these reasons and because the great majority of violence prevention activities occur at the local level, it is important that, whenever possible, federal data collection systems allow for small-area estimation.

There are several models of data collection systems that allow for estimating national, state, and local patterns simultaneously. For example, the Youth Risk Behavior Surveillance System has three complementary components: (1) a national school-based survey, (2) state and local surveys, and (3) a national household-based survey (Kolbe et al., 1993). These three components provide comparable information on risk behaviors in different subpopulations of adolescents in the United States. Another example is the Fatal Accident Reporting System supported by the National Highway Traffic Safety Administration. This system collects detailed information on all fatal motor vehicle crashes in the United States (National Highway Traffic Safety Administration, 1993). The system also links data on these events across police records, medical examiner and coroner files, emergency medical service reports, and hospital medical reports. Because this system is essentially a census, state and local data are easily obtainable. This system has provided extremely useful data for evaluating the effectiveness of state laws designed to prevent motor vehicle fatalities (e.g., safety belt laws, child safety seat laws).

CONCLUSIONS

Violence is a serious problem facing American families and communities. Recognition of the enormous costs of violence in terms of direct medical expenses, psychological trauma, and damage to community institutions is growing. Given the cost of violence to communities, little has been invested in research and data collection that would provide a rational basis for prevention and control. Existing data collection systems that provide information on the incidence, patterns, and consequences of violence suffer from fragmentation, response error, undercoverage, and lack of information about important aspects of the problem.

Coordination at the federal level to measure violence and its consequences would improve the quality, consistency, and efficiency of data collection efforts. Federal coordination would also encourage methodological research on such key issues as improving the validity of responses on sensitive issues, improving the efficiency of screening for violent incidents, capturing the complexity of violent events, improving coverage of persons unconventionally attached to households, and estimating the impact of violence in local areas.

REFERENCES

Biderman, A.D.
1981 Sources of data for victimology. *Journal of Criminal Law and Criminology* 72: 789-817.

Brush, L.D.
1990 Violent acts and injurious outcomes in married couples: Methodological issues in the National Survey of Families and Households. *Gender and Society* 4:56-67.

Bureau of Justice Statistics
1992 *Criminal Victimization in the United States, 1990.* National Crime Victimization Survey Report (NCJ-134126). Washington, D.C.: U.S. Department of Justice.

Cook, P.J.

1985 The case of the missing victims: Gunshot wounding in the National Crime Survey. *Journal of Quantitative Criminology* 1:91-102.

Elliott, D.S.

1994 Serious violent offenders: Onset, development, course, and termination—The American Society of Criminology 1993 Presidential Address. *Criminology* 32:1-21.

Federal Bureau of Investigation

1993 *Crime in the United States 1992.* Available from the U.S. Government Printing Office. Washington, D.C.: U.S. Department of Justice.

1984 *Uniform Crime Reporting Handbook.* Available from the U.S. Government Printing Office. Washington, D.C.: U.S. Department of Justice.

Fingerhut, L.A., and J.C. Kleinman

1989a Mortality among children and youth. *American Journal of Public Health* 79:899-901.

1989b Trends and current status in childhood mortality: United States, 1900-85. *Analytical and Epidemiological Studies.* Series 3, No. 26, NCHS Publication No. (PHS) 89-1410. Hyattsville, Md.: National Center for Health Statistics.

Finkelhor, D., G.T. Hotaling, and A.J. Sedlak

1992 The abduction of children by strangers and nonfamily members: Estimating the incidence using multiple methods. *Journal of Interpersonal Violence* 7:226-243.

Gelles, R.J., and M. Straus

1988 *Intimate Violence.* New York: Simon and Schuster.

Hogan, H.

1993 The 1990 post-enumeration survey: Operations and results. *Journal of the American Statistical Association* 88:1047-1060.

Kolbe, L.J., L. Kann, and J.L. Collins

1993 The Youth Risk Behavior Surveillance System: Overview. *Public Health Reports* 108(Supp. 1):2-10.

Loftin, C.

1986 The validity of robbery-murder classifications in Baltimore. *Violence and Victims* 1:191-204.

Loftin, C., K. Kindley, S.L. Norris, and B. Wiersema

1987 An attribute approach to relationships between offenders and victims in homicide. *Journal of Criminal Law and Criminology* 78:259-271.

Loftin, C., D. McDowall, and B. Wiersema

1992 Economic risk factors for infant homicide. Pp. 273-275 in *Proceedings of the 1991 Public Health Conference on Records and Statistics.* Hyattsville, Md.: National Center for Health Statistics.

McCaig, L.F.

1994 National Hospital Ambulatory Medical Care Survey: 1992 Emergency Department Summary. Advanced data from Vital and Health Statistics (No. 245). Hyattsville, Md.: National Center for Health Statistics.

Mercy, J.A., and L.E. Saltzman

1989 Fatal violence among spouses in the United States, 1976-1985. *American Journal of Public Health* 79:595-599.

Moore, K.A., C.W. Nord, and J.L. Peterson

1989 Nonvoluntary sexual activity among adolescents. *Family Planning Perspectives* 21:110-114.

National Center on Child Abuse and Neglect

1988 Study of national incidence and prevalence of child abuse and neglect, study findings. Washington, D.C.

National Center for Health Statistics
1993 *Vital Statistics of the United States 1989.* Volume II - Mortality, Part A. Hyattsville, Md.: National Center for Health Statistics.

National Highway Traffic Safety Administration
1993 *Fatal Accident Reporting System 1991.* Washington, D.C.: U.S. Department of Transportation.

National Victim Center
1992 *Rape in America: A Report to the Nation.* Arlington, Va.: National Victim Center.

Osgood, D.W., P.M. O'Malley, J.G. Bachman, and L.D. Johnston
1989 Time trends and age trends in arrests and self-reported illegal behavior. *Criminology* 27:389-417.

Poggio, E. C., S.D. Kennedy, J.M. Chaiken, and K.E. Carlson
1985 *Blueprint for the Future of the Uniform Crime Reporting Program: Final Report of UCR Study.* Prepared for the Federal Bureau of Investigation. Washington, D.C.: U.S. Department of Justice.

Robinston, J.G., B. Ahmed, P.D. Gupta, and K.A. Woodrow
1993 Estimation of population coverage in the 1990 United States census based on demographic analysis. *Journal of the American Statistical Association* 88:1061-1071.

Rokaw, W.M., J. Mercy, and J. Smith
1990 Comparability and utility of national homicide data from death certificates and police records. *Public Health Reports* 105:447-455.

Straus, M.A., and R.J. Gelles
1990 *Physical Violence in American Families: Risk Factors and Adaptations to Violence in 8,145 Families.* New Brunswick, N.J.: Transaction Publishers.

Straus, M.A., R.J. Gelles, and S.K. Steinmetz
1980 *Behind Closed Doors: Violence in the American Family.* New York: Anchor Press/Doubleday.

Sweet, J.A., L. Bumpass, and V.R.A. Call
1988 *The Design and Content of the National Survey of Families and Households.* Madison: University of Wisconsin, Center for Demography and Ecology.

U.S. Consumer Product Safety Commission
1986 *NEISS: The National Electronic Injury Surveillance System: A Description of Its Role in the U.S. Consumer Product Safety Commission.* Washington, D.C.: U.S. Consumer Product Safety Commission.

World Health Organization
1977 *Manual of the International Classification of Diseases, Injuries, and Causes of Death* (Ninth Revision). Geneva, Switzerland: World Health Organization.

Appendix

Workshop on Integrating Federal Statistics on Children

conducted by
THE COMMITTEE ON NATIONAL STATISTICS
and
THE BOARD ON CHILDREN AND FAMILIES
NATIONAL RESEARCH COUNCIL
INSTITUTE OF MEDICINE

March 31-April 1, 1994

National Academy of Sciences
Cecil and Ida Green Building—Room 104
2001 Wisconsin Ave., NW
Washington, D.C.

Thursday, 31 March

8:30-9:00 a.m. Continental Breakfast

9:00-10:00 OPENING REMARKS

Miron Straf, Committee on National Statistics
Deborah Phillips, Board on Children and Families
Robert Hauser, University of Wisconsin, Chair

10:00-12:00 SESSION 1: CHILDREN AND HEALTH CARE REFORM

Paul Newacheck, University of California at San Francisco
with Barbara Starfield, Johns Hopkins University

Discussants:
Nicholas Zill, Westat, Inc.
Robert Valdez, Office of the Assistant Secretary of Health

12:00-1:00 p.m. LUNCH

1:00-3:00 SESSION 2: PATTERNS OF ECONOMIC WELL-BEING AND DEPENDENCY

Greg Duncan, University of Michigan (now at Northwestern University) with
Kris Moore, Child Trends, Inc.,
Brett Brown, Child Trends, Inc., and
Jeanne Brooks-Gunn, Columbia University

Discussants:
Gary Sandefur, University of Wisconsin
Donald Hernandez, Bureau of the Census

3:00-3:15 BREAK

3:15-5:15 SESSION 3: CHILDREN AND INTERPERSONAL VIOLENCE

Colin Loftin, University of Maryland with
James Mercy, Centers for Disease Control and Prevention

Discussants:
David Cantor, Westat, Inc.
Michael Rand, Bureau of Justice Statistics

5:30 RECEPTION

6:00 DINNER

Friday, 1 April

8:00-8:30 a.m. Continental Breakfast

8:30-10:30 SESSION 4: THE TRANSITION TO ELEMENTARY SCHOOL

Sandra Hofferth, The Urban Institute (now at University of Michigan)

Discussants:
John Love, Mathematica Policy Research, Inc.
Jerry West, National Center for Education Statistics

10:30-10:45 BREAK

10:45-12:45 SESSION 5: THE TRANSITION INTO THE LABOR FORCE

Aaron Pallas, Michigan State University

Discussants:
Russell Rumberger, University of California at Santa Barbara
Suzanne Bianchi, Bureau of the Census

12:45-1:45 p.m. LUNCH

1:45-4:00 FINAL PLENARY SESSION

PRESENTERS AND DISCUSSANTS

SUZANNE BIANCHI, Population Division, Bureau of the Census
JEANNE BROOKS-GUNN, Center for the Study of Children and Families, Teachers College, Columbia University
BRETT BROWN, Child Trends, Inc., Washington, DC
DAVID CANTOR, Westat, Inc., Rockville, MD
GREG DUNCAN, Center for Urban Affairs and Policy Research, Northwestern University
DONALD J. HERNANDEZ, Population Division, Bureau of the Census
SANDRA HOFFERTH, Institute for Social Research, University of Michigan
COLIN LOFTIN, Department of Criminology, University of Maryland
JOHN LOVE, Mathematica Policy Research, Inc., Princeton, NJ
JAMES MERCY, Division of Violence Prevention, National Center for Injury Prevention and Control, Centers for Disease Control and Prevention, Atlanta, GA
KRISTIN MOORE, Child Trends, Inc., Washington, DC
PAUL NEWACHECK, Institute for Health Policy Studies, University of California at San Francisco
AARON PALLAS, Department of Education, Michigan State University
MICHAEL RAND, Crime Surveys Branch, Bureau of Justice Statistics, U.S. Department of Justice
RUSSELL RUMBERGER, Department of Education, University of California at Santa Barbara
GARY SANDEFUR, Department of Sociology, University of Wisconsin
BARBARA STARFIELD, Department of Health Policy and Management, Johns Hopkins University
ROBERT VALDEZ, Office of the Assistant Secretary of Health, U.S. Department of Health and Human Services
JERRY WEST, National Center for Education Statistics, U.S. Department of Education
NICHOLAS ZILL, Westat, Inc., Washington, DC